makeup makeovers | weddings

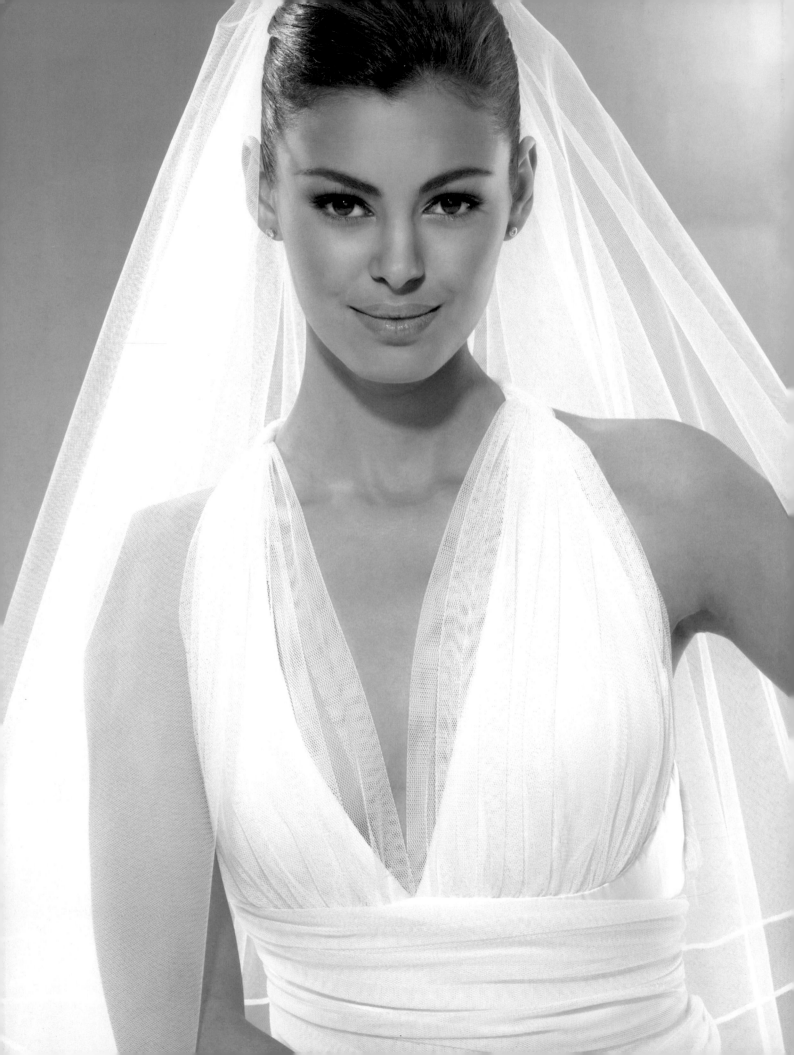

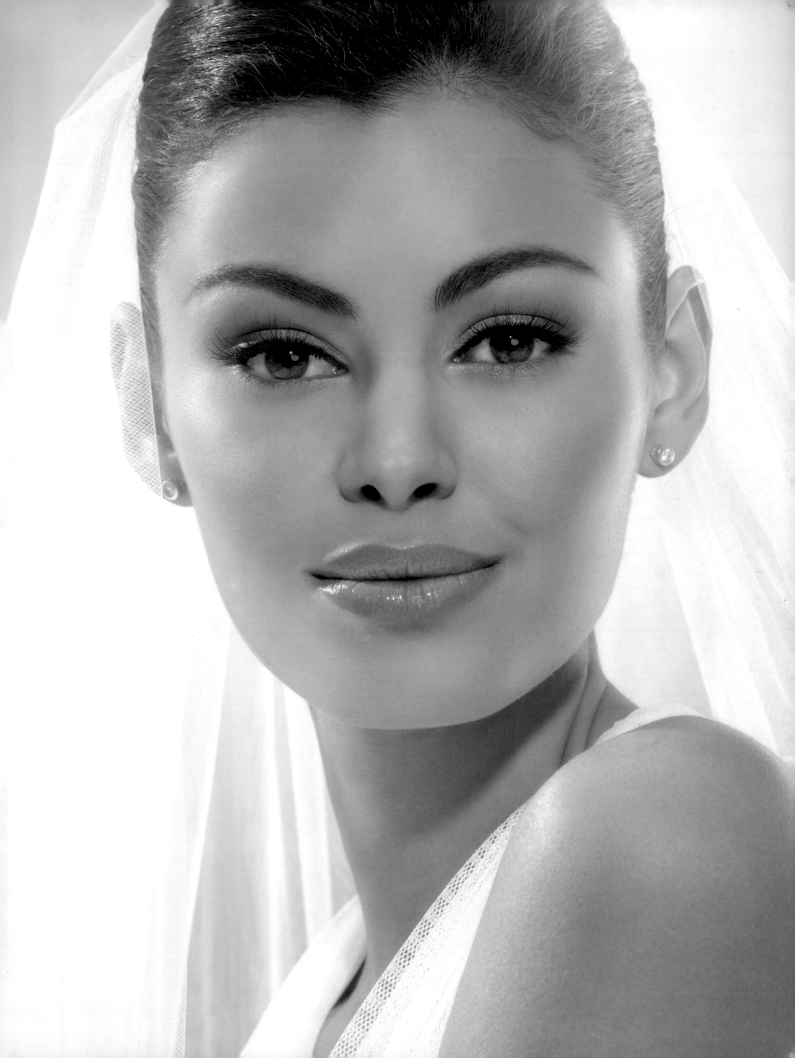

makeup makeovers | weddings

stunning looks for the entire bridal party

robert jones
founder, simple beauté

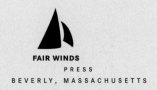

FAIR WINDS
PRESS
BEVERLY, MASSACHUSETTS

Text © 2006 by Robert Jones and Lisa Bower

First published in the USA in 2006 by
Fair Winds Press, a member of
Quayside Publishing Group
100 Cummings Center
Suite 406-L
Beverly, MA 01915
www.fairwindspress.com

10   4 5

ISBN - 13: 978-1-59233-231-1
ISBN - 10: 1-59233-231-5

Library of Congress Cataloging-in-Publication Data available

Text by Robert Jones with Lisa Bower
Book design by Carol Holtz Design
Hair and makeup by Robert Jones, assisted by Susie Jasper, Missy Brumley, and Lisa Williams
Representation by Seaminx Artist Management, www.seaminx.com
Produced by Elaine Moock, Sunni Smyth, and Tiffany Mullen
Fashion and beauty photography by Jeff Stephens
Fashion styling by Chad Curry
Still-life photography by Fernando Ceja
Still-life styling by Phillip Groves
Illustrations by Robin Kachantones
Jewelry courtesy of H2 herrenhuffaker, www.herrenhuffaker.com
Flowers courtesy of M. Bountiful, a flower shop in Dallas
Bridal gowns courtesy of Saks Fifth Avenue, Galleria Dallas, Stanley Korshak in Dallas,
Neiman Marcus, Downtown Dallas, and Myrdith Leon-McCormack in New York
Special thanks to Patty Woodrich for her never-ending support (I could not have done this without her)
and Michael Glassmoyer for his original vision!
www.simplebeaute.com

Printed and bound in China

This book is dedicated to the people who believed
in me, even when I was not sure that I believed in myself:
Chip, the love of my life; Missy, my best friend; Elaine and Sunni,
the rocks that keep me going; and Tiffany and Mike, without whom
none of this would be possible!

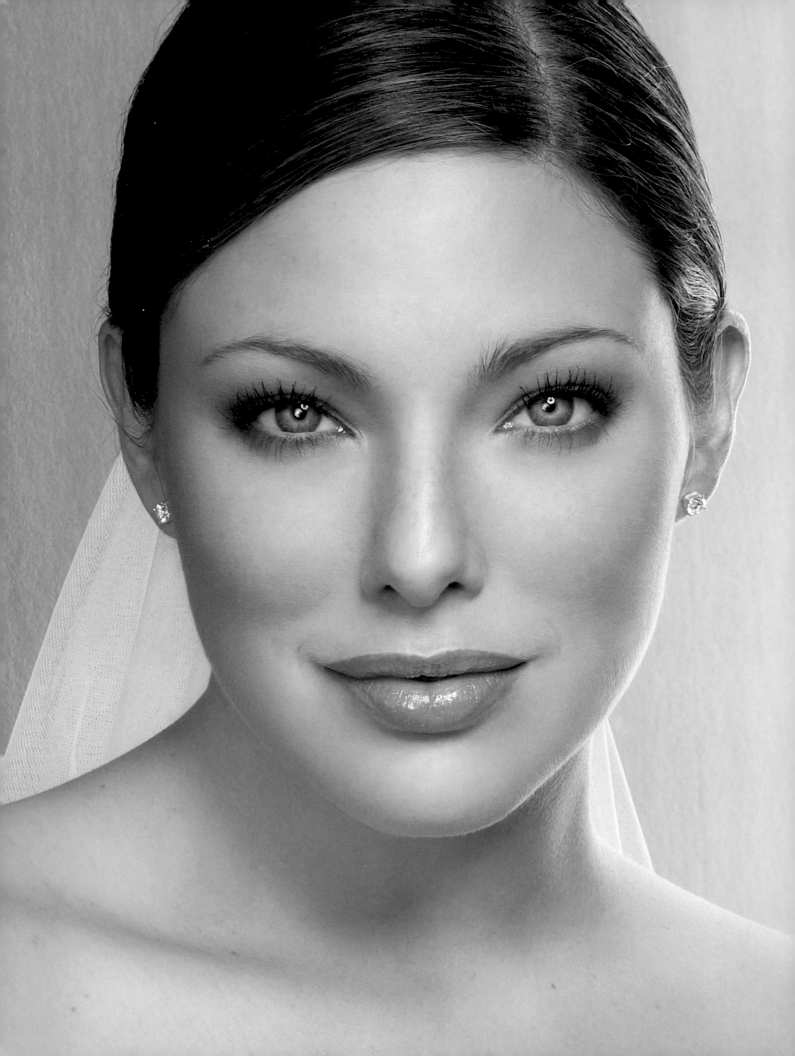

introduction

I know you're excited and ready to experiment with new colors to find the perfect look for your wedding. My makeup tips are intended to make you feel beautiful and confident for one of the most special days of your life.

I also want to emphasize how important it is to remember that makeup is meant to be beautiful, and beautiful makeup is all about the colors you use and where you place them. Makeup should be used to accentuate and highlight your best features—not to cover up or disguise you. Instead of focusing on your flaws, learn how to focus on your best, most beautiful features.

Despite what the magazines show you, there is no such thing as a naturally perfect face. Every face has its own unique features, and the sooner you discover and celebrate yours, the happier and more confident you'll be as you walk down the aisle toward your new life. Just remember, every woman is beautiful!

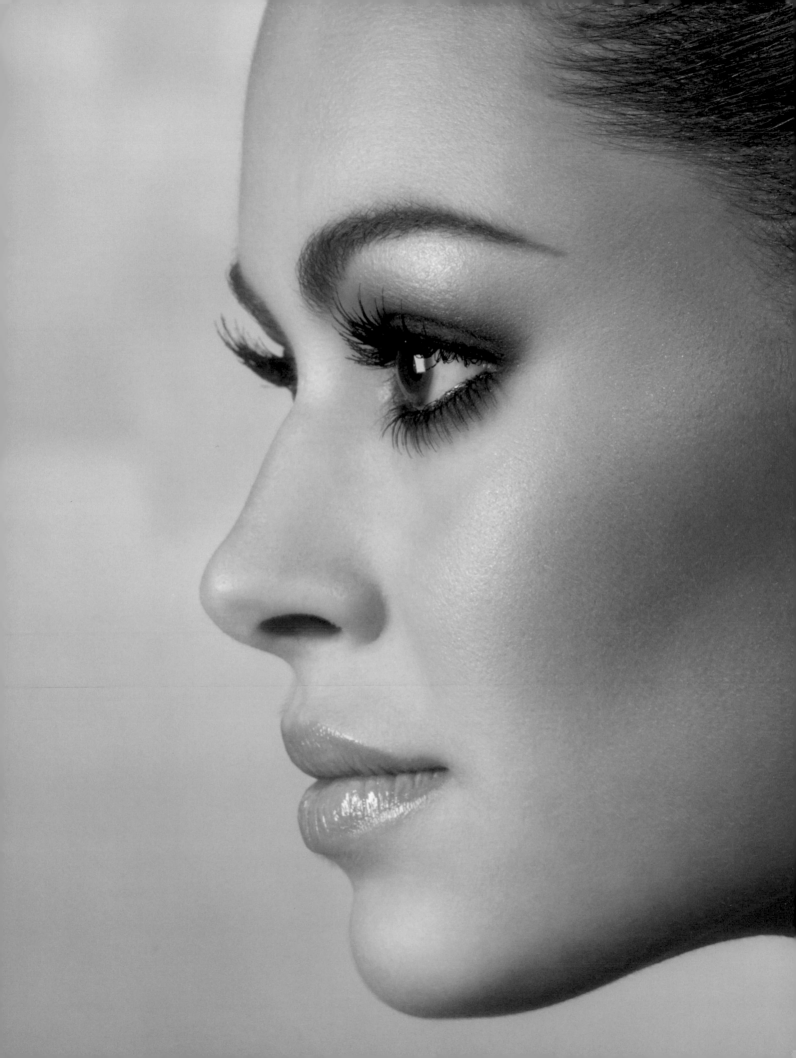

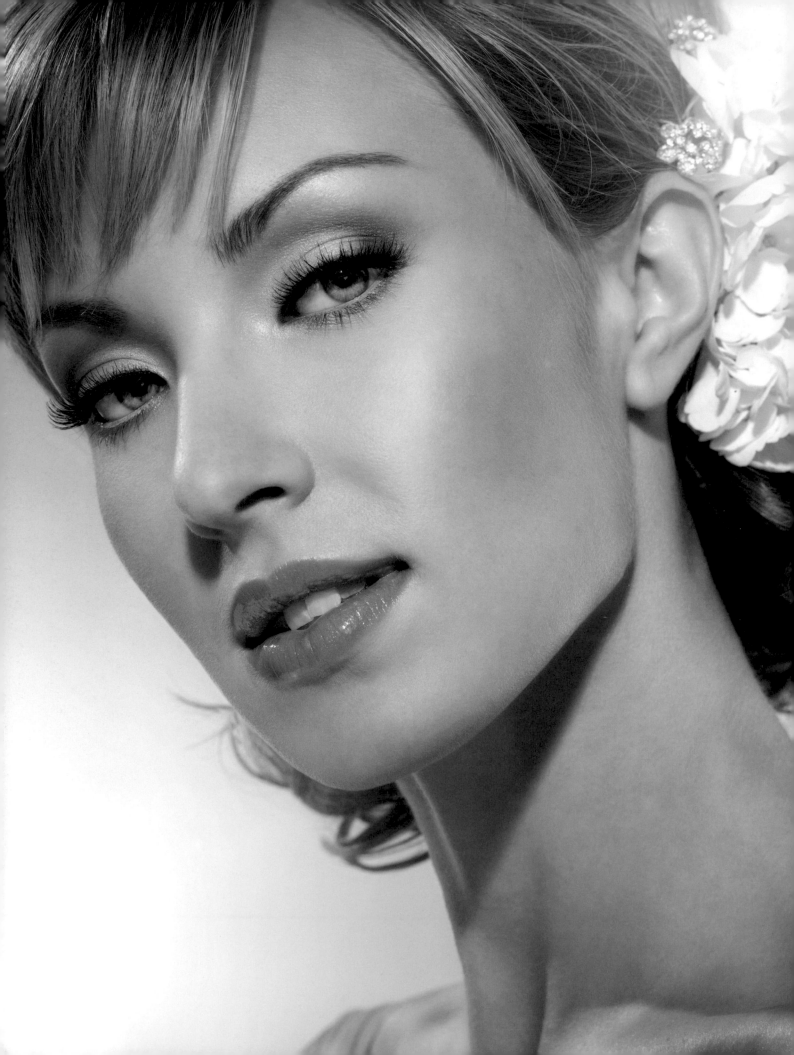

chapter one | introduction to bridal beauty

Your wedding day is so special and exciting. It is truly a day that is just about you and the beginning of the rest of your life. You are about to marry the person that you love and dream of spending forever with. I want to help you make it the most special day of your life.

I have had the pleasure of helping some of the most beautiful women celebrate their wedding day. I count them among the most beautiful not because they were fashion models or famous actresses (although I have made up my share of those), but because they radiated a glow of love and excitement for the future. I feel that I can help you look your most beautiful as well, but first I think we need to briefly discuss what true beauty is.

True beauty is not about being the made-up ideal of the perfect beauty, but instead it is about having self-confidence and loving who you are. True beauty comes from the expression in your eyes and the character in your face. It comes from within, and we are going to bring out your inner beauty and self-confidence.

I think that *every* woman is beautiful; it is just a matter of helping her find her own true beauty. It has been proven that if a woman looks her most beautiful, she will *feel* her most beautiful. This book is all about showing you how to look *your* most beautiful.

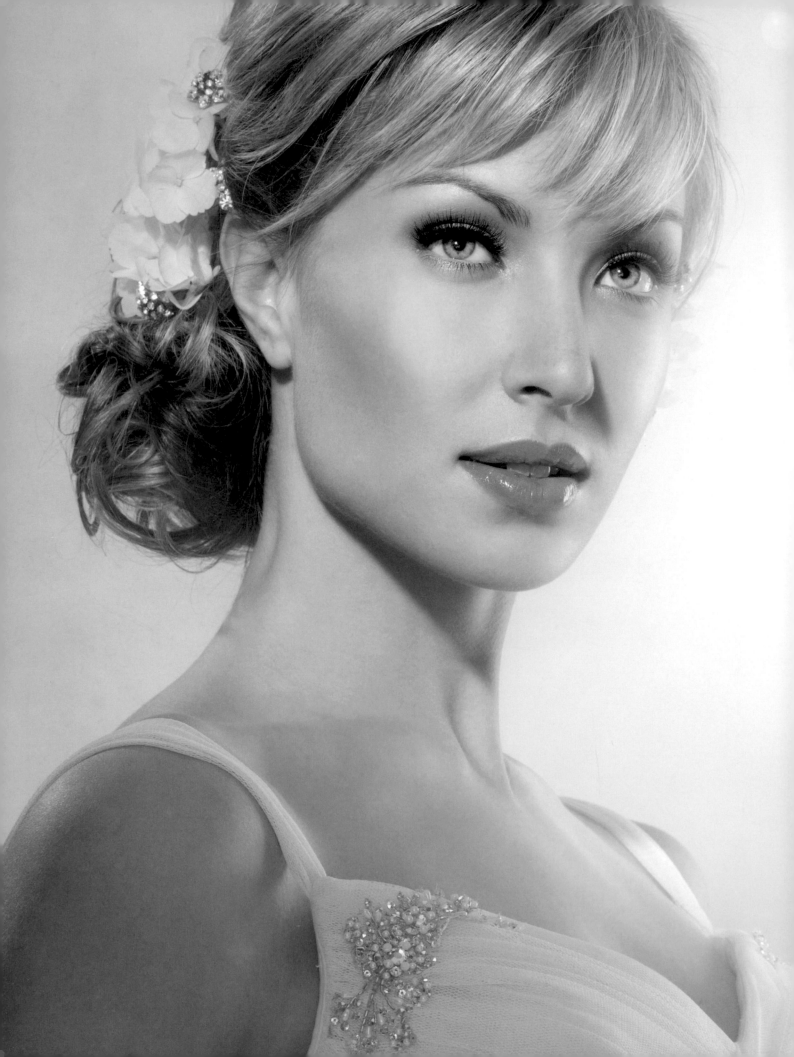

taking your time

When preparing for a wedding, most women spend weeks—even months—choosing the right dress. Then they'll spend weeks trying to find the perfect shoes. And then there's the time spent selecting the wardrobe for the entire bridal party. Many times, the anticipation leading up to the wedding is as much fun as the event itself. I know you would not *dream* of waiting until the last minute to find the perfect wedding dress. Yet that's exactly what many women do when it comes to planning their makeup for the wedding and reception!

I want to make sure you're not one of them. You have to be prepared and ready for your day. It's important to find the perfect look ahead of time. You do not have to necessarily try something completely new, but you should fine-tune your look, and practice applying your makeup. The wonderful thing about makeup is that it will wash off, so feel free to play! If you don't get the look you want, you can always start over.

Lucky for you, you don't have to start from scratch. You were smart enough to get some professional help. By reading all my tips and all the information in this book, you will help yourself be the most amazing you possibly can be. I am so excited that you chose me to help you on your special day!

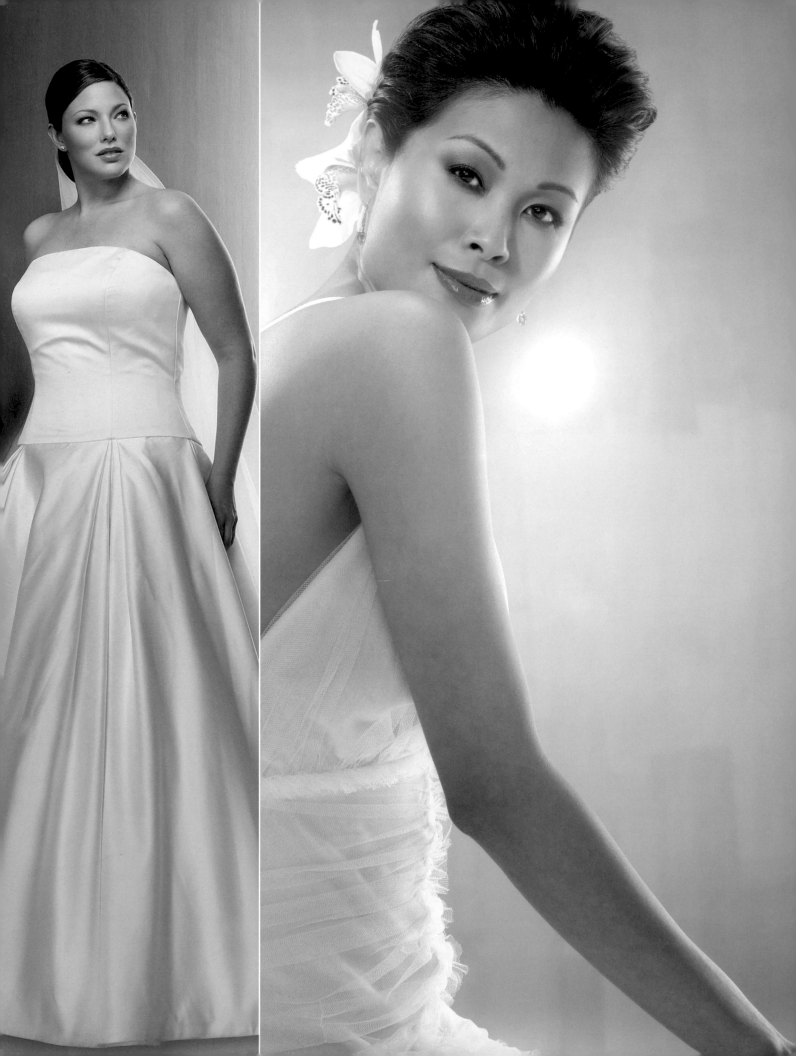

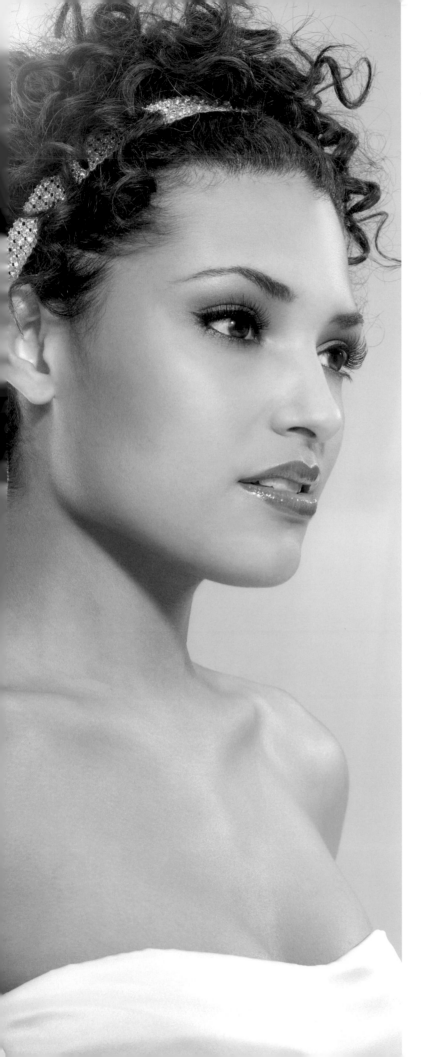

In this book, you'll find:

- Important makeup tips for the bride-to-be
- Correct color choices based on a variety of lighting situations
- Wedding photo and bridal portrait tips
- Application techniques to give you your perfect look
- Makeup tips for your bridesmaids

  And so very much more!

  So read on, and get ready to become the most beautiful bride that you can be!

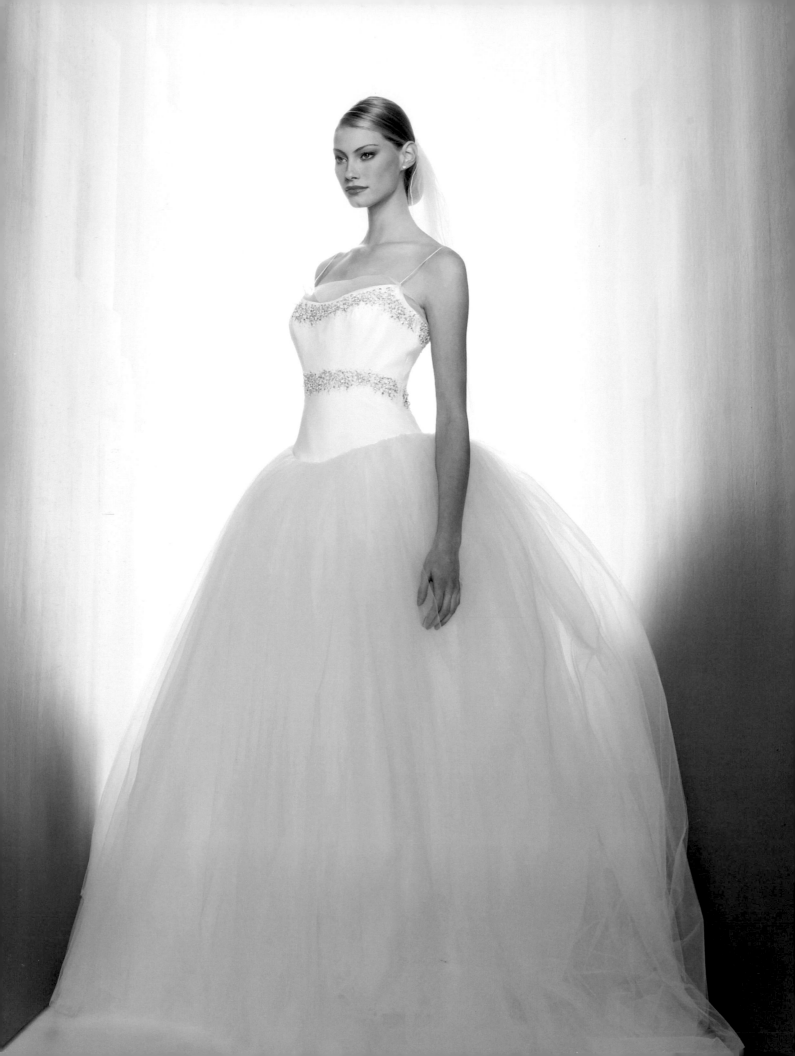

chapter two | # bridal beauty

I believe that choosing the look of your wedding day makeup is as important as choosing your gown. Yet so many women spend months looking for the perfect dress and thirty seconds deciding on the makeup look for their special day. Your look will be captured in photos forever, so it's important to put on your best face with no mistakes. After all, you are the very center of attention on your wedding day. Why leave your look to chance?

This book will help you decide what kind of bride you want to be: a classic beauty, a glamour gal, or a sophisticated bride. With a little planning, practice, and advice from me, you and your entire bridal party can look picture-perfect on your wedding day.

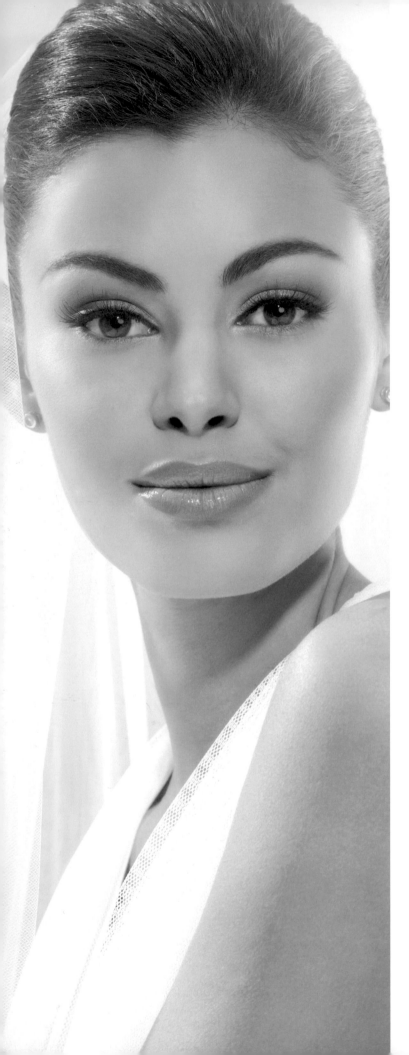

classic vs. trendy

The most important advice I can give you is this: Don't try a new look on the day of your wedding. Try new looks, maybe even several new looks, before your special day. This gives you a chance to see how all the looks appear before the day and to choose the one you really love.

Stay away from extreme makeup trends and go for a slightly more classic look that enhances your best features. You can go with something very modern or nontraditional if you want. You could even wear a color other than white for your special day.

Ask yourself this question: If you or your children were to look back on your wedding portrait and all the other photos fifteen years from now, would you still think you look pretty? That's a good rule of thumb to follow to decide if the makeup and hair looks you're choosing will stand the test of time.

Just make sure that, on your wedding day, you still look like you. You don't want to change your whole look so that people don't recognize you. Trust me, you don't want to overdo it and pile on the makeup. It is important to look like yourself—just the most beautiful you possible.

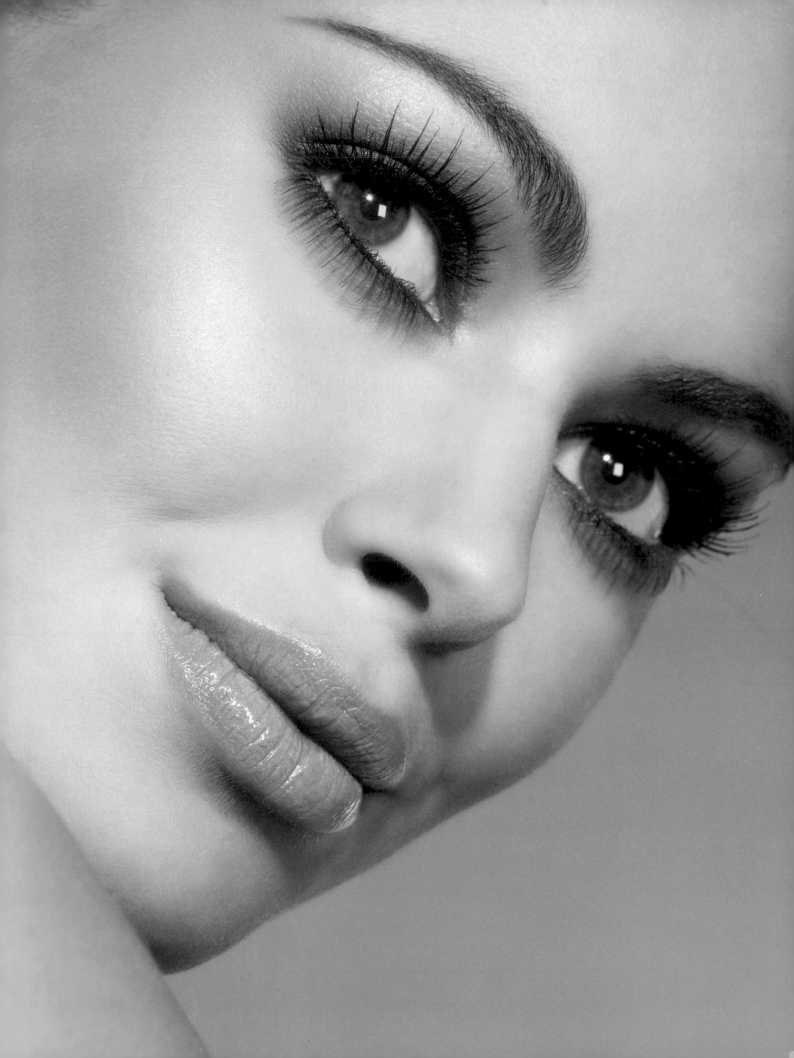

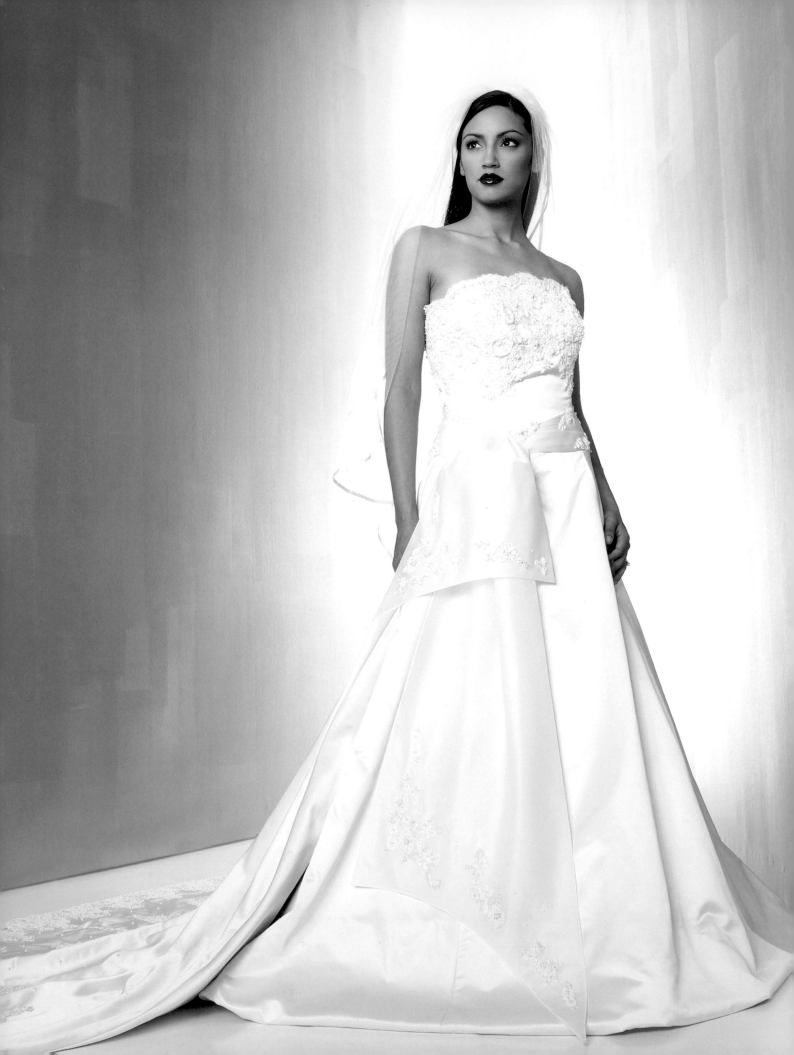

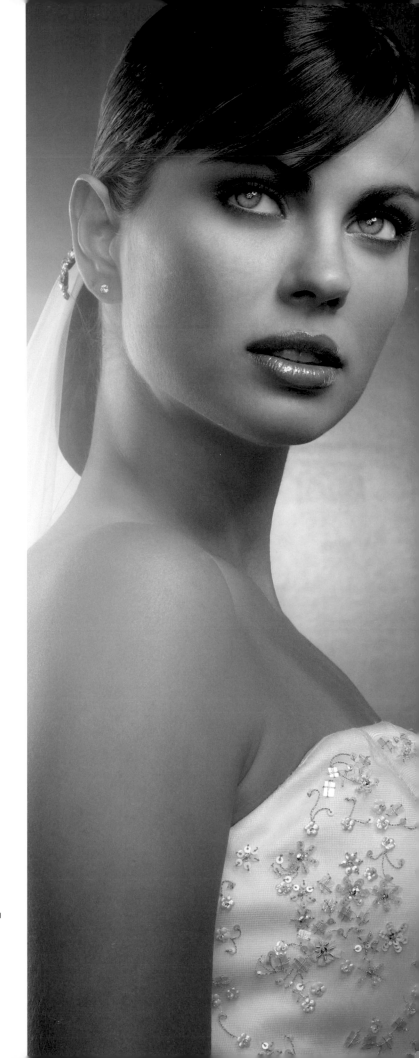

picture perfect

Here is another essential piece of advice: While you are trying new looks (*before* your wedding day, remember!), photograph them. I love to use a Polaroid camera, with its immediate gratification, but you could use a digital or disposable camera—whatever you have.

You will learn so much about what you have done and how each little change you make will photograph professionally. (I know that is hard to believe, but it's true.) Plus, it's fun! You could even make a party out of it: invite your bridesmaids over and have them do the same thing. I always take advantage of any reason to have a party!

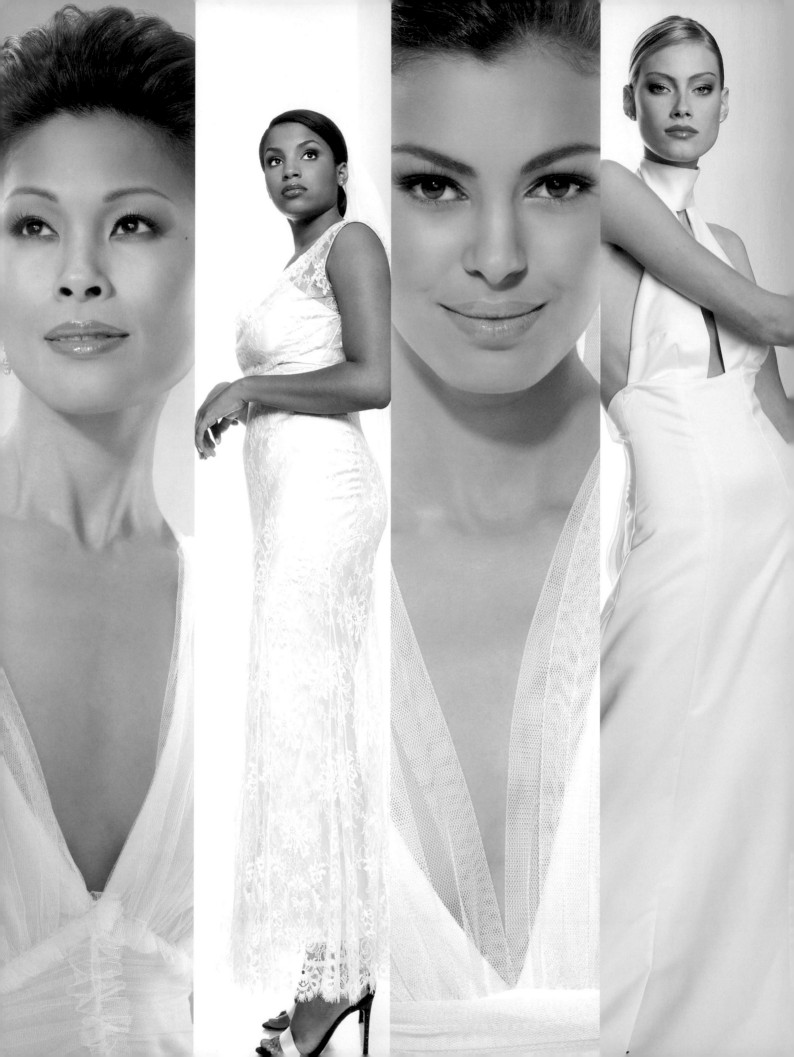

chapter three | perfect timing

The time of day for your wedding will affect your makeup choices. A more natural look for a morning wedding varies greatly from the more dramatic look of an evening ceremony. The way the sunlight changes throughout the day can influence the way your makeup appears in photos. It can also affect the type of lighting your photographer will choose when he or she photographs you.

I divide brides into four categories, based on the time of day they're getting married: morning, midday, late afternoon, and evening. With each time choice, there are certain details you'll want to consider. Paying attention to these details can help you get the look, and the wedding photos, of your dreams.

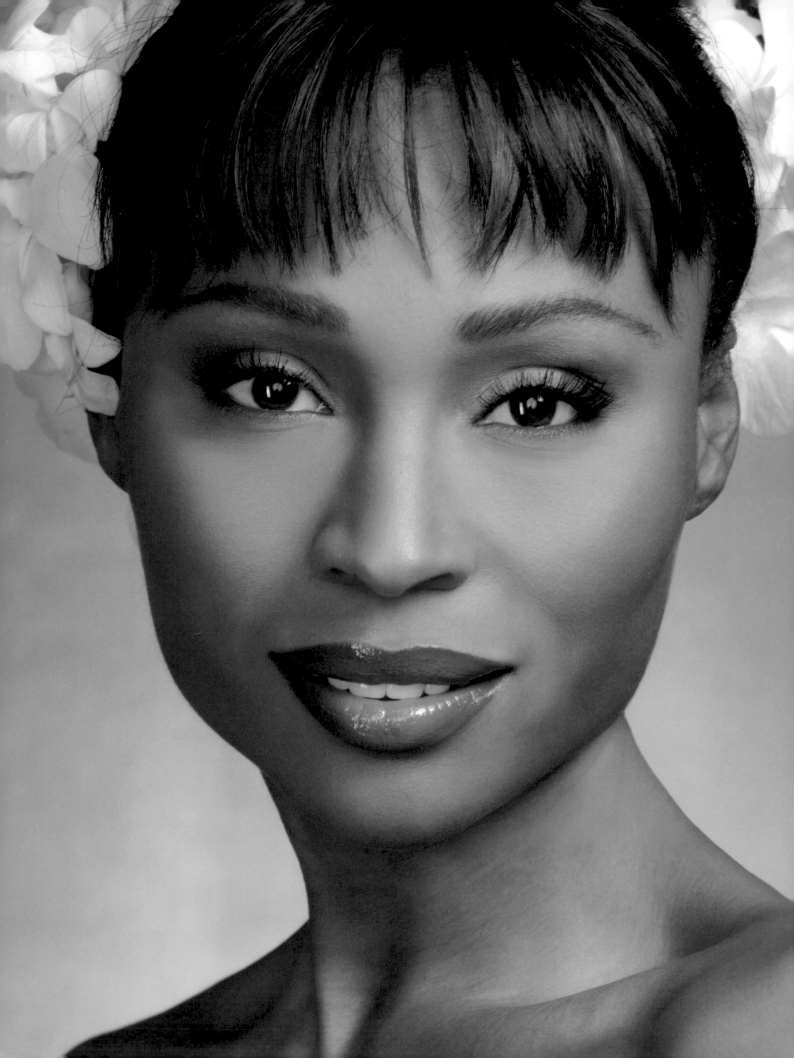

morning bride

If you're planning a morning wedding, your makeup look should appear soft and pretty to match the cool, soft morning light. Mornings are perfect for the natural girl, because it's the time of day when a bride should wear the least amount of makeup. I find that most brides who are getting married in the morning are having the event outside, or at least taking their photos and portraits outside. Even if they are getting married inside, the photographer will be taking advantage of the natural light coming through windows rather than a lot of artificial light for the photographs.

- Though a matte foundation is always perfect for photographs, a morning bride can choose to wear a foundation with a slight sheen or dewiness to it, because the light is so soft. Make sure that your skin is a nice, even tone. For the perfect application that will last all day, see page 37.

- If your skin tends to break out, I would not choose this time of day for your wedding, because you are going to want to wear as little foundation and concealer as possible due to the softer natural light.

- Go light on the powder so your face retains its natural appearance. You want your skin to appear matte, but it does not take a lot of powder to achieve this. Heavy powder can appear artificial, especially in the morning light.

- Do not make bold eyeshadow color choices for your eyes if you are having a morning wedding. Choose warmer, soft shades that complement your eye color. This is the one time you will want to wear less eyeshadow, because the lighting will accentuate any harsh colors or lack of blending.

- Make sure to define your eyes really well at the lashline to help them stand out. To learn how to get the most from your mascara for great definition, see page 61. Another option would be false eyelashes; turn to page 62 for simple, foolproof application instructions.

- If you choose to wear eyeliner (you do not have to wear any) make sure to keep it subtle and soft. You do not want anything too dark (no black) or too harsh (not too thick—keep it really close to the lashline) at this time of day.

- Lip color should always be soft and natural— nothing too bold at this time of day. If it is too bold, it will be all you see in the photos.

- Everything will photograph darker than it appears to the eye, because the light is so soft, so go with softer shade choices.

- Bridesmaids' dresses should be in a soft color, and bridesmaids should also wear softer makeup shades.

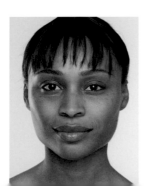

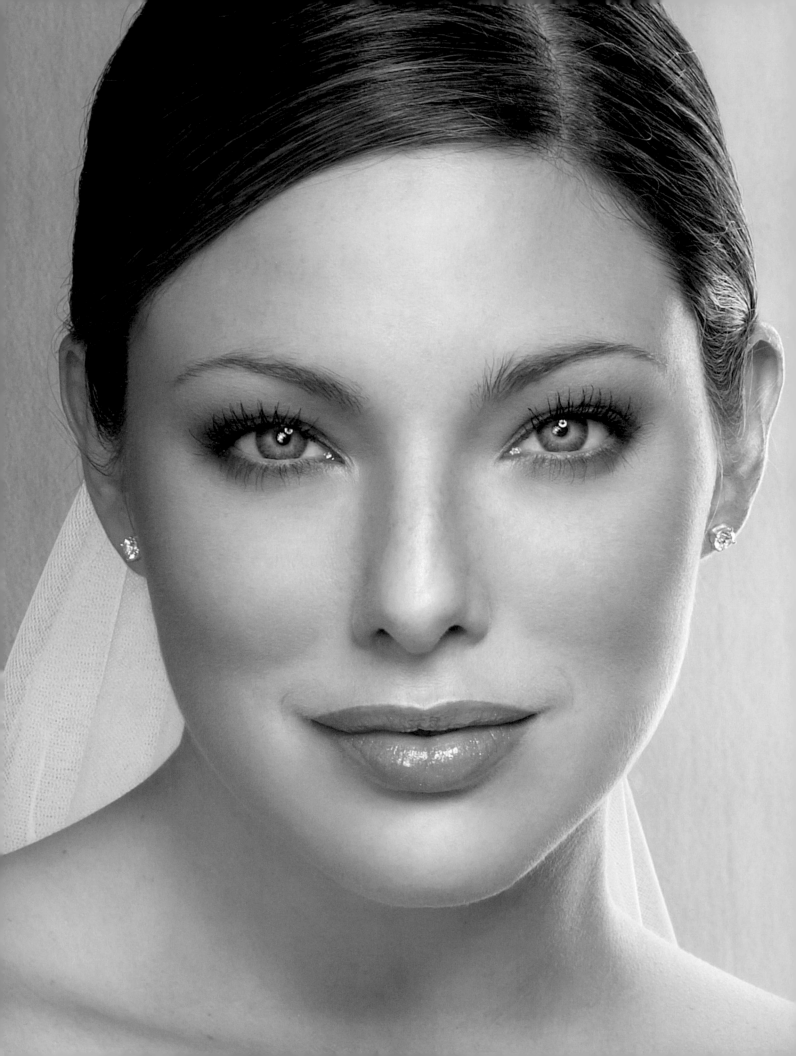

midday bride

If you're planning a wedding in the middle of the day, be aware that the midday sun can cast shadows on your face, which can make a difference if you're taking outdoor photos. This is the harshest light to be photographed in. Since natural light is directly above you at this time, you'll want to follow these steps to make sure you are "picture perfect."

- Do not wear foundation with a sheen or dewiness to it. If there is any sheen to the face, it will look too shiny and reflective in the photographs. This is a time when you will want to wear the least amount of foundation possible, because it will show the most. A lightweight foundation and a matte powder finish will photograph beautifully.

- Make sure your blush has a more matte finish, too. If it has too much shimmer, it will also look too shiny in the photos.

- A crème blush is a great choice for this time of day. It will absorb into your skin and look more natural. Keep in mind that crème blush does not work well on oily skin—stick with a powder blush if you fall into this category.

- Due to the midday lighting, if your eye makeup is too dark, your eyes will look like two dark holes in your photographs. Your highlight shade is the most important shadow choice at this time of day. Use a highlight with shimmer (not frost) to open up the eyes. The light-reflective particles in the shimmer will help prevent the "black hole effect." Make sure your midtone and/or contour shade has a matte finish—you never want to use three shades with shimmer, because the eye will look too shiny in the photographs. See page 79 for the perfect natural eyeshadow application process.

- If you want to wear eyeliner, keep it as close to the lashline as possible. If it is too thick, it could darken the lid more than you want, creating the dreaded "black hole effect."

- Long, beautiful lashes really help define your eyes without depending on heavy eyeliner. To learn how to get the most from your mascara, see page 61. False eyelashes would also be a perfect choice; turn to page 62 for foolproof application instructions.

- Since the sunlight grows stronger as midday approaches, every makeup line becomes more visible. Make sure to blend your foundation, blush, eyeshadow, and powder very well. At this time of day, there is no such thing as overblending.

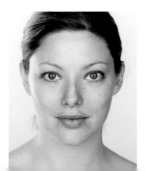

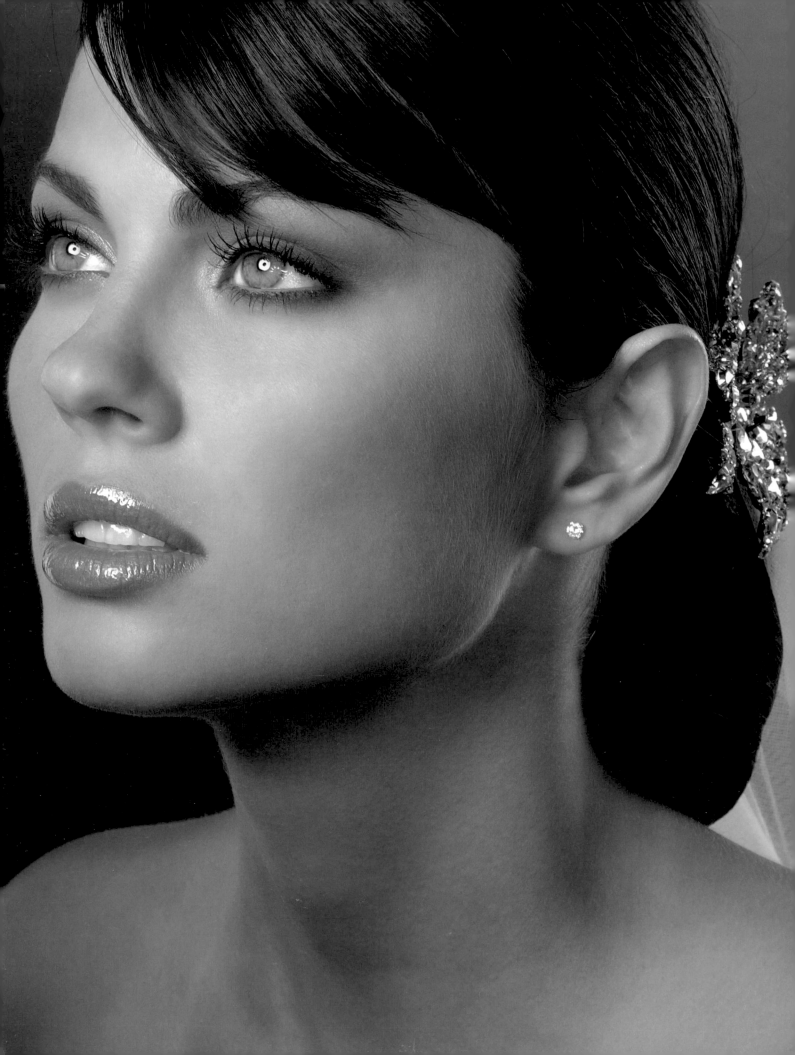

late-afternoon bride

The golden light of late afternoon is the most beautiful light you can be photographed in. Late afternoon is when the sun is starting to set in the sky, creating a beautiful warm glow. Since the light is so beautiful and forgiving, you can add a little more drama to your makeup look. The light is growing softer and warmer, so you can wear more eyeshadow and have more shade options.

- If your skin is less than perfect, late afternoon is a great time to get married. The light is softer and more forgiving, so you can use a little more foundation and concealer to cover your flaws, and your skin will still appear completely natural looking in photographs. Don't forget to powder— remember that matte skin always photographs better than shiny skin.

- As evening comes, your photographer will have to use a flash, so make sure you add color to your face. A flash shoots a bright burst of light at your face, which can make you appear washed out. Even if you do not normally wear blush on a daily basis, you need to wear at least a little color on your cheeks. I promise, you will not look or photograph like you belong on a street corner if you wear a soft bit of color on your cheeks! Another great way to prevent looking too

pale or washed out in your photos is to contour your face and add a warm glow with bronzing powder. To learn how to contour or "sculpt" your face, see page 90.

- It's fine for your blush to have shimmer in it, because it will look beautiful in this light, though it is also perfectly fine if you want to use a shade that is matte.

- You can make richer color choices because of the forgiving lighting. So feel free to apply more dramatic eyeshadow shades.

- A shimmery (not frosted) eyeshadow will look beautiful at this time of day, because it photographs well in all lighting. Just make sure that your midtone and/or contour shade has a matte finish. You never want to use three shades with shimmer, because the eye will look too shiny in photographs.

- Want to add a little more glamour? Try false eyelashes. This is the perfect time of day for this beauty trick, and lashes help define your eyes better than anything else you could do. Turn to page 62 to find out how to apply them. If you don't want to wear false lashes, then just make sure to layer your mascara to get the most definition you can. Turn to page 61 for layering techniques.

- Late-afternoon brides get the green light to wear a richer lip color, too. The light allows you to wear richer colors, since they won't show up in photos as too intense.

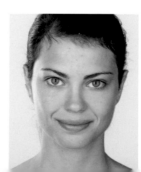

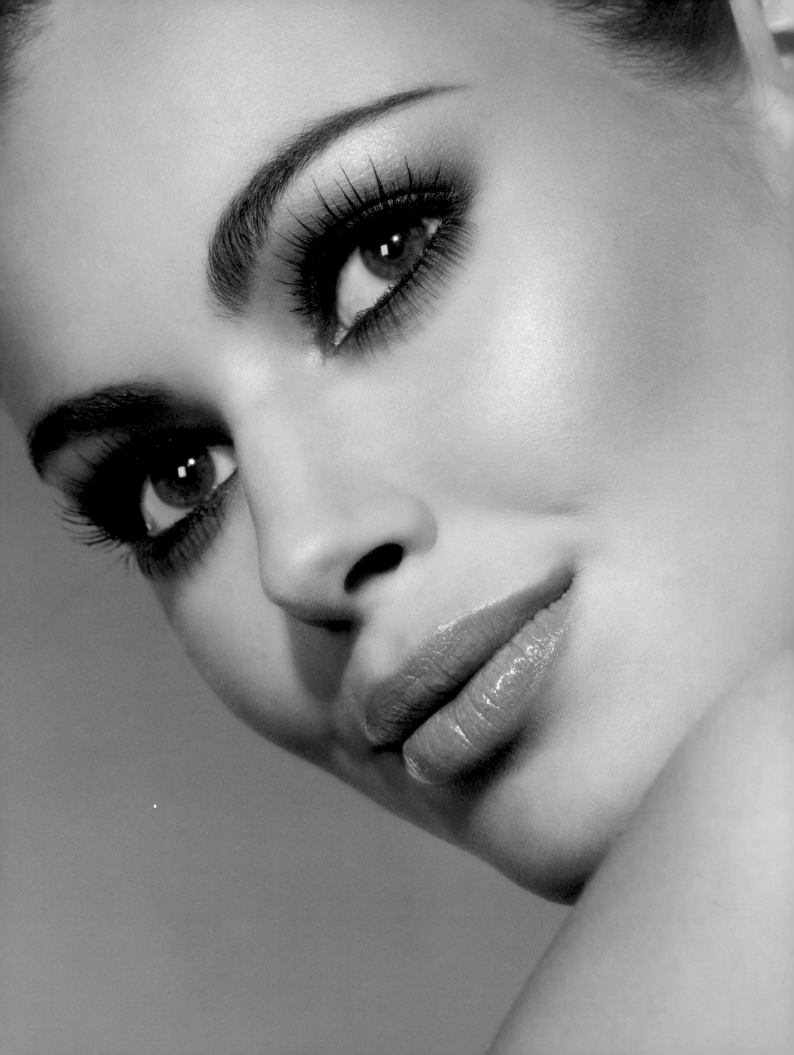

evening bride

If you love to glam it up, an evening wedding allows you to go for a more dramatic makeup look. You can play with color and wear more makeup than at any other time and still photograph beautifully. This is the time of day for the bride who wants to be a glamour queen. Remember that every photograph will be taken with a flash, which definitely makes a difference in your choices.

- If you have less than perfect skin, this is a great time for you. You can wear more foundation and powder and still look natural.

- Make sure to bronze generously to give your skin a glow. One thing that helps is "sculpting" your face, because it will add color so the flash will not wash your skin out, and it adds dimension. Dimension is important because the flash can also flatten everything out in a photograph. Turn to page 90 to learn how to use makeup to sculpt your face.

- Everything should be more defined—from your lips to your eyes to your cheekbones—because all photos will be taken with a flash, which, as I've mentioned, can wash you out. However, more defined does not mean darker. For instance, some women do not wear blush on a daily basis, but you need at least a little color in your cheek because of the flash. Make sure to give your lips a nice defined edge by lining; turn to page 72 for perfect application instructions. Also

for some women, especially natural blondes, even if you may not wear brow color on a daily basis, you may need a little so that your brows will show in the photos. Turn to page 52 for details on applying brow color.

- Shimmery eyeshadow will photograph well for evening, but you should wear absolutely no frosted shadows for this time of night (or any time for brides, in my opinion). Frosted eyeshadow will look too shiny in photos, especially when a flash is used! A shimmery shadow always looks soft and pretty. Just make sure that at least one of your three shades of shadow is matte. You never want all three shades to shimmer, because the eye will look too shiny in your photos.

- In my opinion, false eyelashes are a must for a nighttime wedding, because they help define the eyes really well. Just remember that every picture will be taken with a flash, and the more definition you have at your lashline, the better you will photograph. Turn to page 62 to find out how to apply false eyelashes. Not to worry if you do not want to wear false lashes, turn to page 61 to learn how to layer you mascara for maximum length and volume.

- If a smoky eye look is one you are interested in wearing, evening is a perfect time for this eyeshadow application technique. Learn how to apply it on page 83. Just make sure to wear a soft lip color if you're wearing a smoky eye.

- Make sure you have lip color and powder on at all times. You never know when the camera will flash!

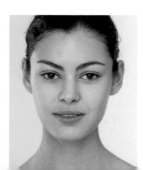

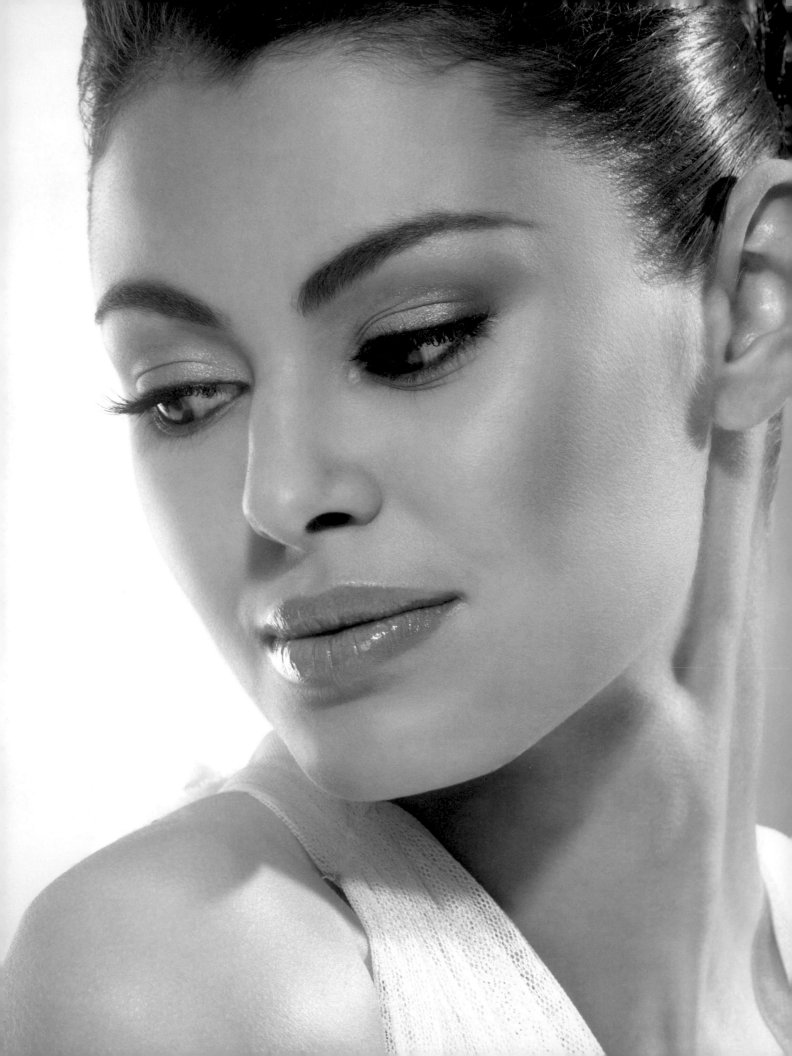

chapter four | perfect application

The key to your wedding day makeup is to apply it so the color lasts throughout the whole event. I want you to have to touch up as little as possible. I do *not* want you worrying about your makeup instead of having fun! I'll show you some little tricks you can do that will allow you to touch up less on your big day.

Bear in mind that applying your makeup for the event is not a matter of wearing heavier makeup. It's more about choosing the right shades and applying color correctly so it will last and look great under several kinds of lighting, from daylight to twilight to your photographer's lights. Throughout this chapter, we will discuss how to create a perfect look for you. I'll tell you how to apply every type of makeup. So read on, and together we can make you look absolutely beautiful—and make your makeup last for the entire event.

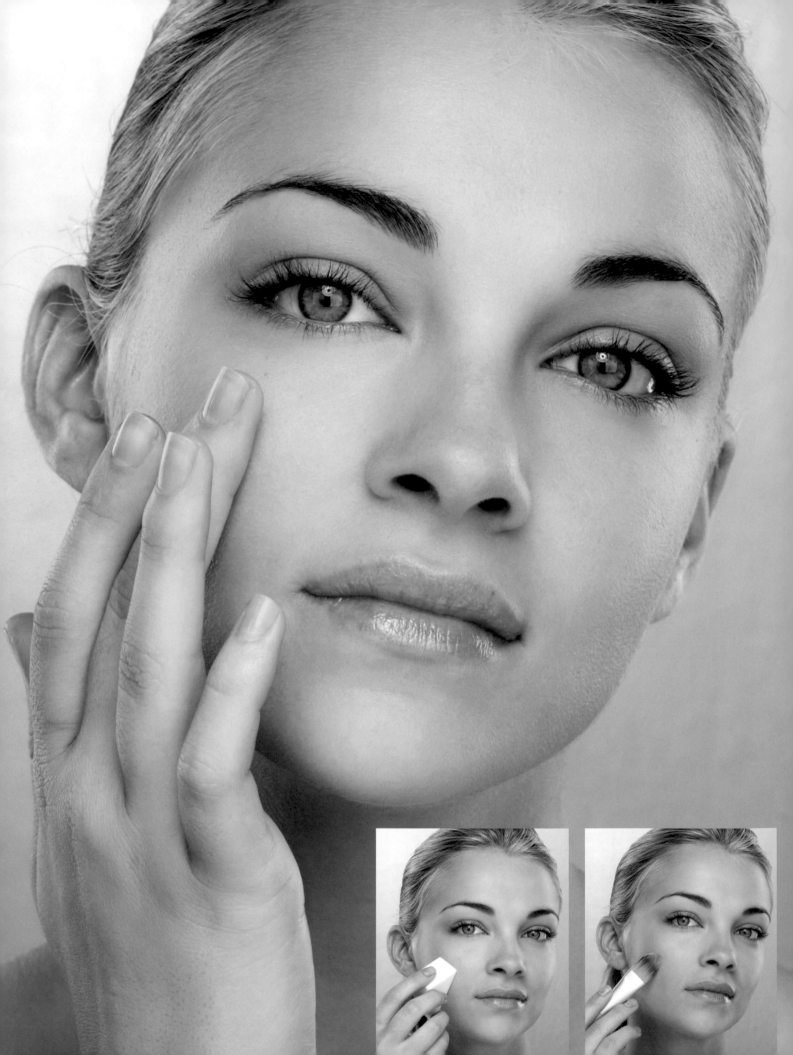

face

Every bride wants beautiful, flawless skin on her wedding day. To ensure this, you'll want to establish a good skincare routine at least two months before the ceremony. This will give your skin a chance to adjust to the new products, so your skin will appear healthy, smooth, and clear. Remember that you will want to experiment and select your makeup look in advance, practicing it several times before the actual wedding date. And don't forget to photograph yourself in your new makeup to get a preview of how you will look in photos.

On the day of the wedding, start your look by applying moisturizer and letting it completely dry. I recommend applying a primer next before applying foundation. Primer is an optional makeup step that can do wonders for your skin's appearance. It helps your foundation go on more evenly and makes it last longer. Next, use concealer to cover up any of nature's imperfections. Then apply a foundation shade as close to your skin tone as possible. When applying foundation, you have three basic tools at your disposal:

- A makeup sponge, which is very sanitary, because you can wash it after each use or throw it away. Sponges also really help with the blending process and help you apply your foundation so it looks smooth and flawless.

- A foundation brush blends foundation well, so it gives you great, even coverage. You should always wash your sponge or your brush after every application. The cleaner the tool, the better the application.

- Don't have a brush or sponge handy? No problem, because the third tool is your finger-

tips. Just make sure to wash your hands after you've applied your moisturizer and treatment products and before you apply your foundation. The residue from the treatment products can compromise the integrity of your foundation and diminish the amount of coverage it provides.

It's best to begin your application in the center of your face, dotting foundation on the cheeks and the forehead, then blending outward. Always remember to finish by blending downward to make sure all the small facial hairs lie flat. After application, blot with a tissue to absorb any excess foundation and moisture left from the product, especially around the nose and in your T-zone (forehead, nose, and chin—all the areas that get shiny first). This will really help with staying power. Even though applying powder will set your foundation and absorb the excess moisture, blotting first will enable you to go longer before you have to touch up.

Finally, using a powder puff or powder brush, add a generous dusting of loose powder to your face to set your foundation for the day. This will help it last longer and give your skin a smooth, even appearance. Make sure your pressed powder compact isn't far away at the wedding and reception for touch ups. Well-powdered matte skin photographs much better than shiny, dewy skin. It's also a good idea to blot your skin with blotting papers or a tissue before reapplying your powder; if you don't, it could create a muddy effect. A helpful tip: Keep your pressed powder in your groom's jacket pocket—by the time you need it, you will be with him, and you will always know where to find it.

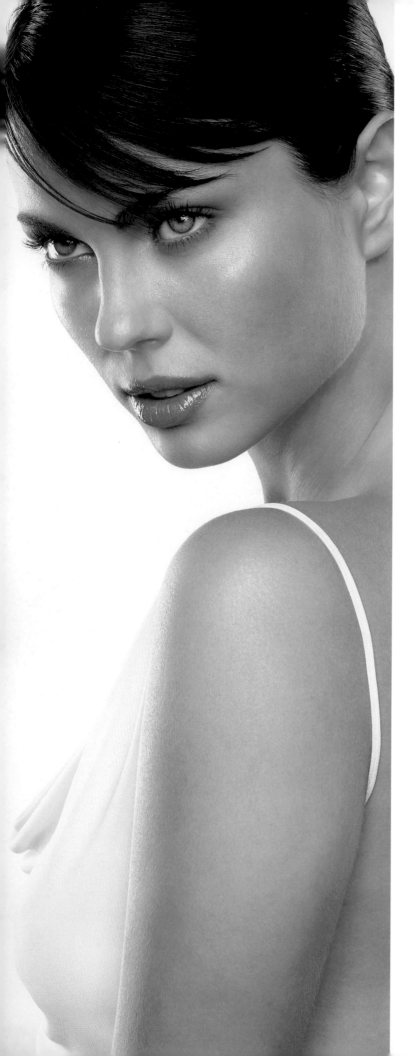

sunless tanning

Because some photography can wash out the skin, you may want to apply a self-tanning lotion to your face and body, starting a few weeks before the wedding to make sure you achieve the shade you want. Make sure you slowly build your color over time to make it appear more natural. Here is the best way to achieve smooth, even coverage when applying self-tanning lotion:

1. Exfoliate well.

2. Moisturize your skin to even out its porosity (your skin's ability to hold moisture).

3. For the body: Mix two parts self-tanner with one part moisturizer. Make sure to pour the self-tanner and moisturizer into a bowl and mix them completely together before you start. Do not try to mix the two in your hands as you apply it—the solution will not go on evenly. If you are very fair, you might want to mix one part self-tanning lotion with one part moisturizer to make it even more subtle.

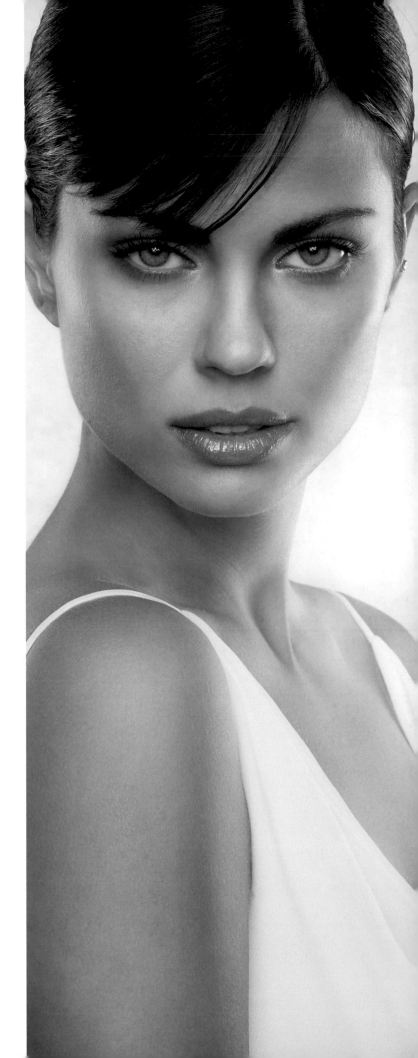

4. For the face: Mix equal parts self-tanning
    lotion with moisturizer to dilute it, and apply
    it to your face over a period of days. If you
    are very fair, you might want to mix two parts
    moisturizer with one part self-tanning lotion
    to make it even more subtle. I recommend
    doing this gradually over a period of time
    instead of in one application, so your skin
    will get a slow build-up of color and appear
    more natural. If you have any dark spots,
    apply some petroleum jelly or a very thick
    moisturizer to the spot before you apply
    the self-tanning lotion; this will prevent
    the spot from taking color or darkening
    as the rest of your skin tans.

Bronzing powder is also a good choice. It can
add warmth to your skin and give you a healthy,
happy glow in your photographs. It is also much
easier to apply, and you do not have to start
weeks in advance. But bronzing powder is only
good for adding color to your face. You do not
want to try to bronze your whole body with
a powder bronzer! It will just make a big mess
by rubbing off on your dress.

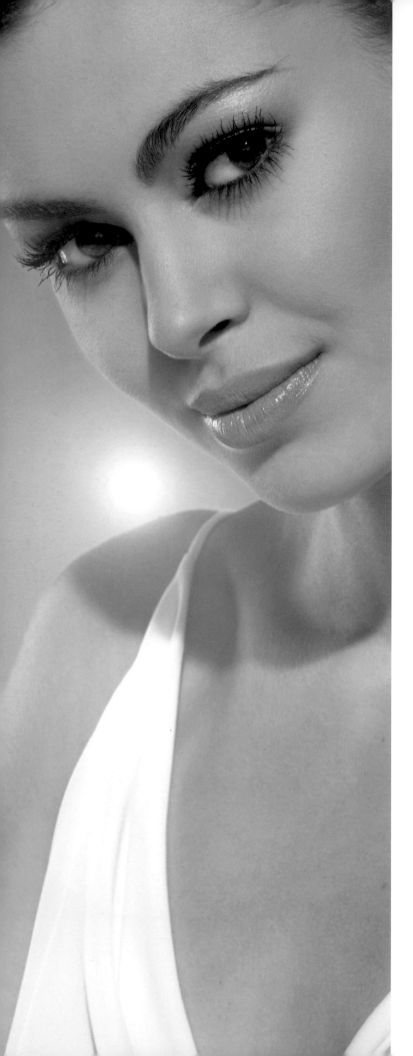

concealer

I already mentioned that we need to conceal any skin imperfections. Let's face it: Very few women have perfectly flawless skin. Yet many women are obsessed with perfection! Everything from sun damage to genetics can affect the surface of your complexion.

Concealer can improve your skin's appearance dramatically, but only if it's invisible. The secret to concealing everything that you do not want to see is applying concealer just to the discolored skin (learning to color within the lines, just like when you learned to color as a child). This is why a concealer brush is so important.

You will actually need to choose different textures of concealer, depending on what you are concealing. Fortunately, there are many different concealers with different textures to help you tackle your problem areas and help your skin look its best.

Remember that concealers are very different from foundations. They are drier, more heavily pigmented, and they "grab" powder differently. If there is an area that you have heavily concealed, it is best to use a lighter shade of powder on this area. If you use the same shade of powder as on the rest of your face, the concealed area may appear darker.

Here are instructions on how to conceal small flaws that might occur.

DARK CIRCLES

To cover undereye discoloration (caused by blood vessels that appear blue or gray when they reflect light), you need to choose the perfect shade and texture of concealer. If you use a formula that is too moist, it can "travel," slipping into creases and fine lines and drawing attention to what you don't want people to notice. A formula that is too dry is bad for the delicate skin around the eyes and can draw attention to those same flaws, and it can appear dry and caked. You might need to experiment to find the perfect formula for you.

You should choose the same shade of concealer as your foundation, or a shade or two lighter if you have truly dark undereye circles. If you're using a concealer that matches your foundation exactly, you may apply it either before or after your foundation. But if you're using one that is lighter, it is best to apply it first.

HERE'S WHAT TO DO:

First, prepare the area underneath the eye by applying eye crème and letting it soak in for two or three minutes. Blot away any excess with a sponge or tissue. Using eye crème will help your concealer adhere, and if the skin under your eyes tends to be dry, your concealer won't "cake up" and call attention to itself. Remember, the undereye area contains fewer oil glands than anywhere else on your body, so it needs plenty of moisture. Be generous with your eye crème, because it's next to impossible to "over-moisturize" this area.

Next, take a concealer brush and apply concealer along the line of demarcation—where the discoloration begins on your skin. Extend the concealer up and over the discolored area. You never want to apply the concealer below the line of demarcation. If you do, you will lighten skin that is already the correct color, and you'll be back where you started—with two uneven shades of skin. Next, take your finger and, using a stippling motion (a patting motion), pat the concealer along the line of demarcation to blend it in. Be sure to conceal any darkness in the corners of your eyes or eyelids, if necessary.

Serious dark circles call for serious concealer. Use a shade or two lighter than your foundation and apply the concealer before your foundation. After you have applied your concealer, and you're applying your foundation, be sure to stipple the foundation over the concealed area. Be gentle—you don't want to wipe away the makeup you initially applied!

Yellow concealers are a great choice for covering very dark circles on ivory and beige skin. And golden-orange concealers work great for covering dark circles on bronze and ebony skin. Both concealers can counteract all shades of skin discoloration, from red to purple to brown.

UNDEREYE PUFFINESS

As painful as it is to admit this, you cannot improve the appearance of undereye puffiness by swiping a light concealer under the eye area. Anything we highlight or lighten on the face makes it stand out more. Our goal is to disguise the puffy area—not make it more prominent!

Instead, you can outsmart the puffy area by highlighting the area just underneath it. Because in most lighting situations (outside, in buildings, and at home), our faces are lit from above, the puffy area creates a shadow on the face. By highlighting the shadowy area, you will bring it out and make the puffiness recede. Because most people look directly at you and not from above, your puffiness will appear even with the rest of your skin. Voilà—you're flawless!

To apply, take a highlighting pen (this is a product designed to specifically highlight recessed areas of the face) or a concealer brush and a light-colored concealer, and apply it just underneath the puffy area right where the shadow is being created. Then lightly blend it with your finger by stippling all along where you applied your product. If you have dark circles as well as puffiness—which many women do—you'll want to use this three-step application:

1. Apply concealer to your dark circles.

2. Next, apply your foundation to your entire face.

3. Now, take your highlighting pen and apply it into the recessed area that is being shadowed by the puffy skin. After this application, make sure to stipple all along the area where you applied your highlighting pen to blend it in.

BLEMISHES

To minimize facial blemishes, you'll want to use a dry-textured concealer so it will cling better to the blemish and not irritate the skin or initiate more breakouts. Apply your foundation first. Make sure you choose a concealer that matches your skin exactly. (A light concealer will only make the blemish seem larger.) Using a concealer brush, apply the concealer directly to the blemish. Then take your finger and stipple to blend the edges around the blemish into the skin.

BROKEN CAPILLARIES OR VEINS

Here, as always, it's important to apply concealer only to the areas of discoloration. You can take a brush and actually draw a line of concealer on top of the broken capillary or vein. Then stipple out the edges to blend. After you have concealed the capillary or vein, apply your foundation over your entire face. When applying foundation over concealer, make sure you stipple it rather than wipe it, so you do not remove your makeup and uncover what you just concealed.

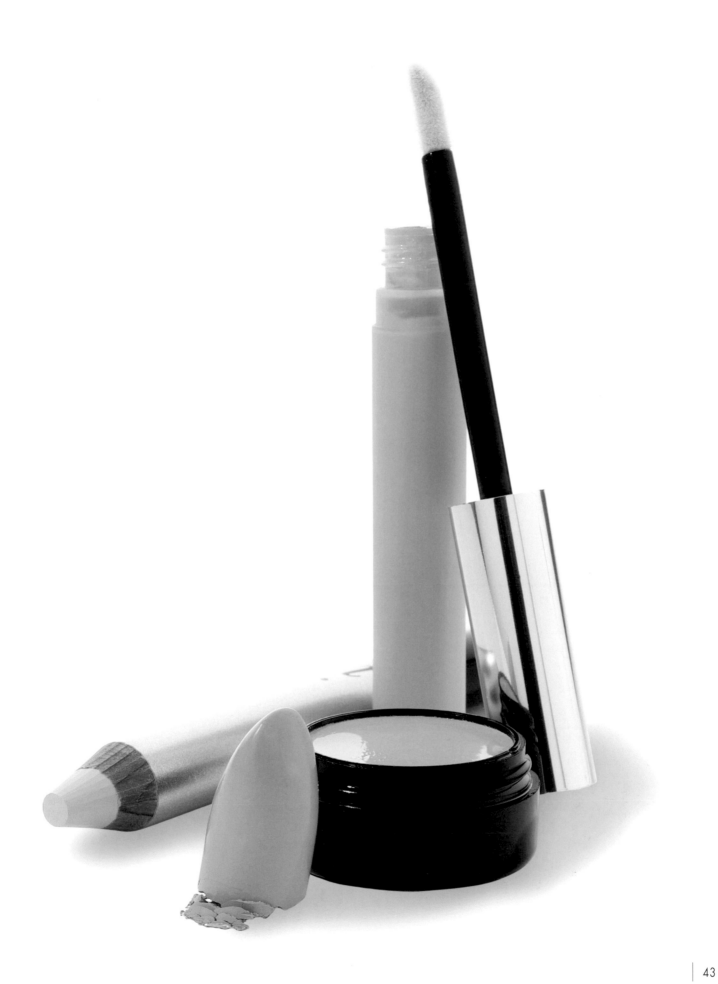

ROSACEA

To counteract the redness of rosacea, you should use a yellow-based concealer, and apply it only to the reddened areas of your face. Then stipple the outer edges with your fingertips, and gently blend the concealer into your skin. Do not overblend, or you will remove all the concealer off of the reddened area. Finish by stippling your foundation over the area, so it will match your skin tone exactly.

HYPERPIGMENTATION OR MELASMA

The terms hyperpigmentation or melasma are the technical terms for brown spots or dark spots on the face. They can be caused from sun exposure or a shift in hormones (such as during pregnancy or with menopause.) These conditions can happen to women with any skin tone. To correct it, you'll want to apply concealer only to the areas that are discolored. Otherwise, if you extend the concealer past the line of demarcation, you will lighten skin that is already the correct color. After applying, you'll want to stipple the edges to blend the concealer. Finish by stippling foundation over the area so it will match your skin tone exactly.

Women with ivory and beige skin tones should use an intense yellow concealer. If you have bronze or ebony skin tones, you should use a golden-orange concealer. The intense undertones of these concealers will help counteract the skin discoloration.

SCARS

A scar is a raised area of skin that has no pores, which makes it difficult to conceal, because pores are what makeup clings to. To conceal a scar, apply a drier-textured concealer directly onto the scar with a concealer brush. Then stipple the edges to blend it in. If you don't have a dry concealer for scars, try this application technique: Apply moisturizer to the scarred area, followed by a bit of loose powder. The moisturizer gives the powder something to cling to. Then take your concealer brush and apply concealer right onto the scar. The concealer and the powder mix together to form a drier texture that will stick better to the scar.

For acne scars, which create texture variation, the best way to make the skin look perfectly flawless is to keep it as matte as possible. Loose powder is your best friend, because it will do just that for you. The last thing you will want to do is to try to fill in the "valleys" by applying too much foundation and concealer.

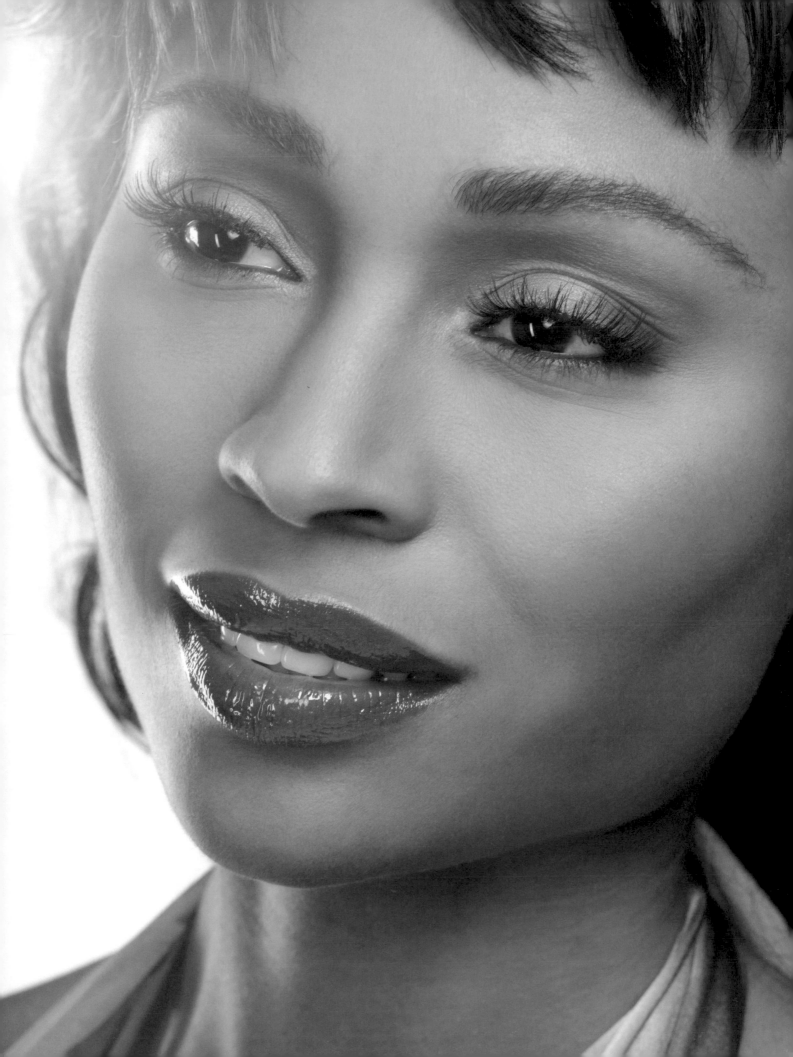

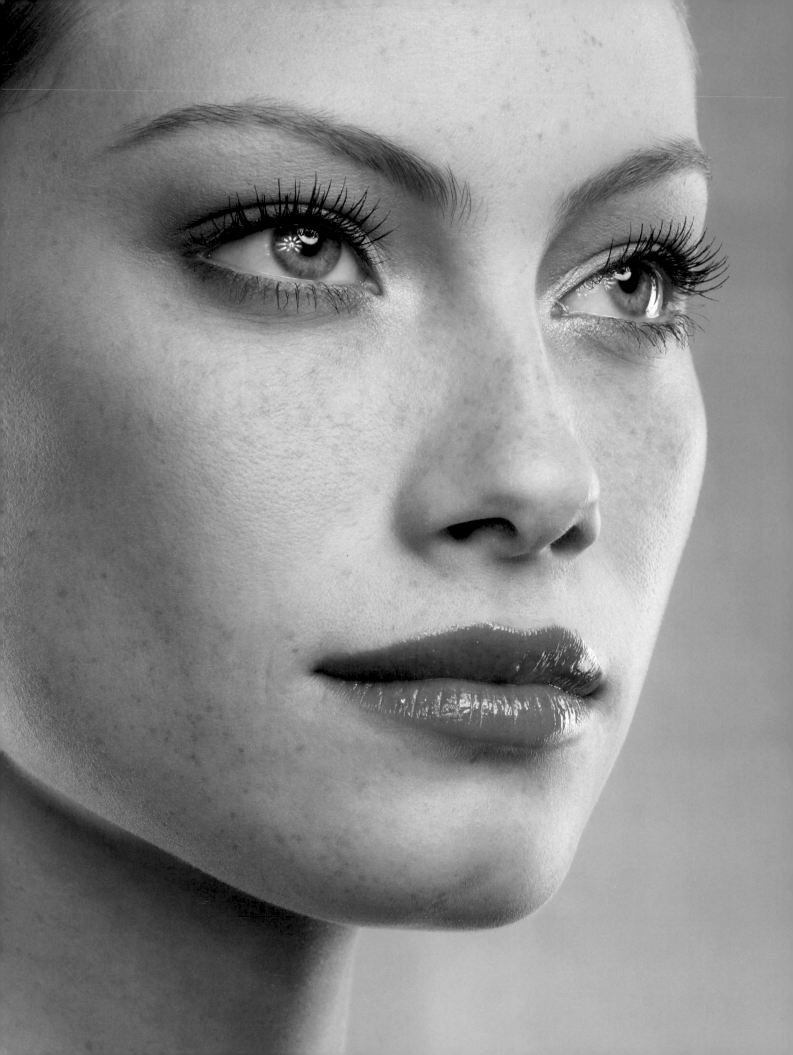

powder

Powder is a makeup must. It sets your foundation; polishes your look; and adds a smooth, velvety softness to the skin. Because loose powder contains more oil absorbers, I prefer to use it to set the foundation, then use pressed powder for touch-ups throughout the day. There are several ways to apply both types of powder:

- A makeup sponge works well for tight areas and is great for "spot" powdering.

- A powder brush is the easiest and most commonly used tool. It is great for blending, but you must be careful not to overblend and brush off what you apply. For best results, apply a little bit of powder at a time (instead of applying it all at once) to ensure smooth, even coverage.

- A powder puff offers the best coverage and is my favorite way to apply powder. Press a puff or sponge into the powder, and then "roll" it onto the skin. Pushing it into the skin with this technique makes your foundation and powder appear as one with your skin and looks far more natural. To finish, lightly sweep the face with a powder brush, using gentle downward strokes to remove any excess powder.

- A fingertip works well for a light powder application. It's a great way to powder underneath the eyes, especially for mature women. Just dip your finger in loose powder. Rub your finger in the palm of your hand to brush off the excess, then trace your finger over the area underneath the eyes to set your concealer and help minimize fine lines.

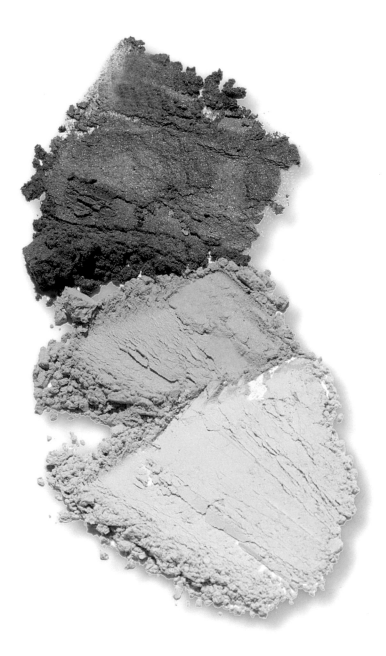

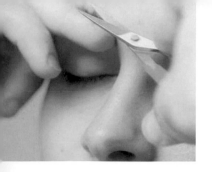
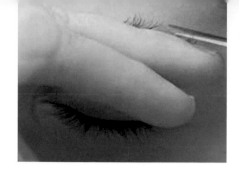
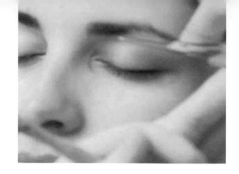

brows

Well-groomed eyebrows are a must. But before you reach for the tweezers, please take some professional advice: You should embrace your natural brow shape, because no matter how much you tweeze, you cannot turn your brows into something they are not. Some brows naturally curve into a gentle arch; others grow straight across. However your brows grow, you need to shape them to suit the way they grow on your face. But never fear! Whatever their shape, you can groom them to flatter your features.

Let's begin by evaluating your brows.

First, are they too dense? Eyebrows that are too dense can be softened either by trimming them or lightening the color.

TRIMMING

To trim your brows, simply brush them up, and snip any stray hairs that extend past the upper brow line. Next, brush them down, and snip any unruly hairs that extend past the lower brow line.

Often, brow hairs are actually longer than they appear, because the tips of the hairs are light in color, and when they reach a certain length, they tend to curl. By trimming them, you trim away some of the density and that slight curl so that the hairs lie down more neatly.

It's important to remember that if you need to trim your brows, it should be done before you start to tweeze. Otherwise you might ruin your brow line by tweezing away hairs that should have stayed but were simply too long.

TWEEZING

Now it's time to tweeze.

The best time to tweeze your brows is after a steamy shower. It's a lot less painful because your pores are already open. Try to tweeze in natural light. You can see what you're doing much better.

If you do what I call "tweezing side to side" it will help you tweeze your brows more evenly. Very few women have brows that grow identically on their face. What this means is that you could tweeze one brow into the shape you want, but because of the way they grow, you couldn't make the other brow match the first one no matter how you tweezed.

Instead, start by tweezing a couple of hairs out of one brow, then switch to the other, tweeze a couple out of it, then switch back to the first, so you'll avoid this problem. By doing this each time you switch brows, you have to re-evaluate what needs to be tweezed, and by comparing that often it will help you get them more even. Always tweeze in the same direction as the hair grows, or the hair might not grow back properly.

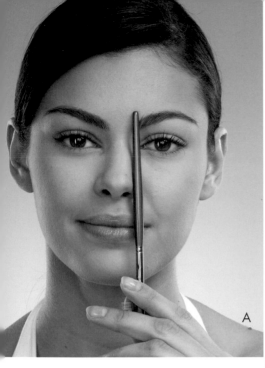

HOW DO YOU DETERMINE WHERE TO START?

By locating three key pivotal points of reference, we will know where and what to tweeze. Simply follow these directions and you will have perfect brows.

POINT A. Hold a pencil or the handle of a brush vertically against the side of your nose, noticing where it meets the brow. That is where your brow should begin.

POINT B. Hold the pencil against your nostril and move it diagonally across the outer half of the iris of your eye. Notice where the pencil meets the brow: This is the best place for the peak of your arch. If you tweeze from Point A to Point B, tapering the line slightly thinner toward the peak, you will create the ideal shape for your brow.

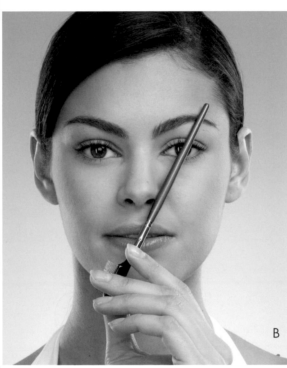

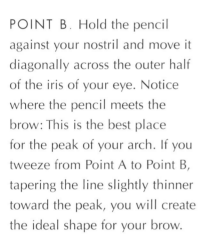

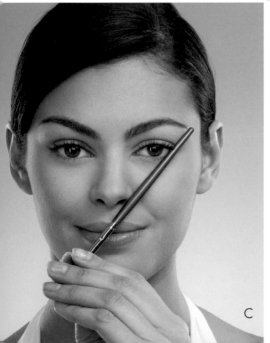

POINT C. Again, place the pencil against your nostril, but this time, extend it diagonally to the outer corner of your eye. Where it meets the brow is the best place for your brow to end. If you tweeze from Point B to Point C, tapering the line even thinner, you will create the best brow shape for your face.

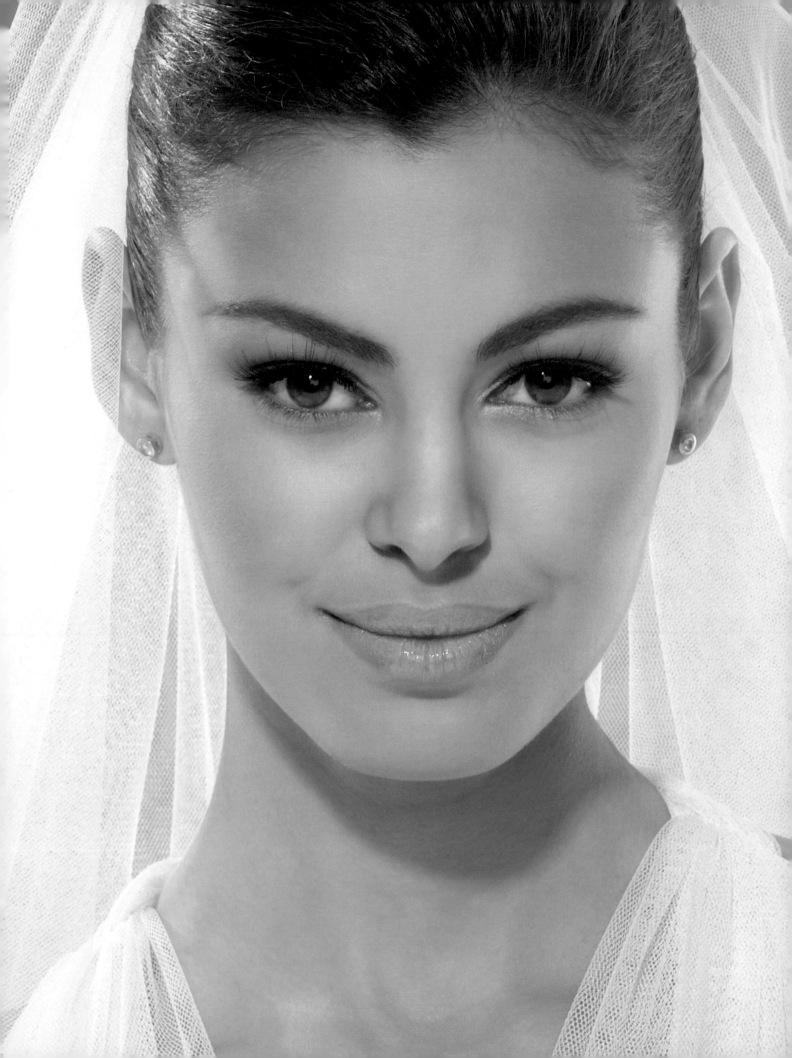

brow color

When selecting a brow color, choose one that is either your natural brow color or one shade lighter. Be careful not to confuse brow pencil and brow powder with eye pencil and eyeshadow—they are not the same!

Brow pencils are duller in color, usually have no sheen, and have a somewhat waxier texture than eyeliner pencils do. Eyebrow powder is duller and more matte than eyeshadow.

When using a brow pencil, apply it in short, feathery, hairlike strokes angled in the same direction as your brow hairs' natural growth.

Never draw on a solid, hard-looking line. Short, feathery, hairlike strokes are meant to imitate short brow hairs. I like to go over the area again, using a small, angled brow brush, following the same stroke pattern. This blends the pencil in a little better and helps it appear more natural.

You can also achieve a very natural brow by using brow powder. Apply it with a small, stiff, angled brow brush in short, feathery strokes, while following the natural hair growth pattern. Remember, you are trying to imitate brow hairs.

For those with scars or brows that are just not there, you may need more coverage. The best way to get a lot of coverage is to layer brow pencil and brow powder on at the same time. First, apply your brow pencil, then simply layer the brow powder directly on top of your pencil strokes. Layering these two products will give you the absolute maximum coverage and will help your color last longer.

FINISHING TOUCHES

Whichever method you prefer, always finish by using a toothbrush-shaped brow brush to brush upward and outward. This will assure that your brow hairs are lying in place and will blend your color beautifully to give you an absolutely natural effect. If you like, you can end with a brow gel. It acts like hairspray for the brows, keeping all the hairs in place.

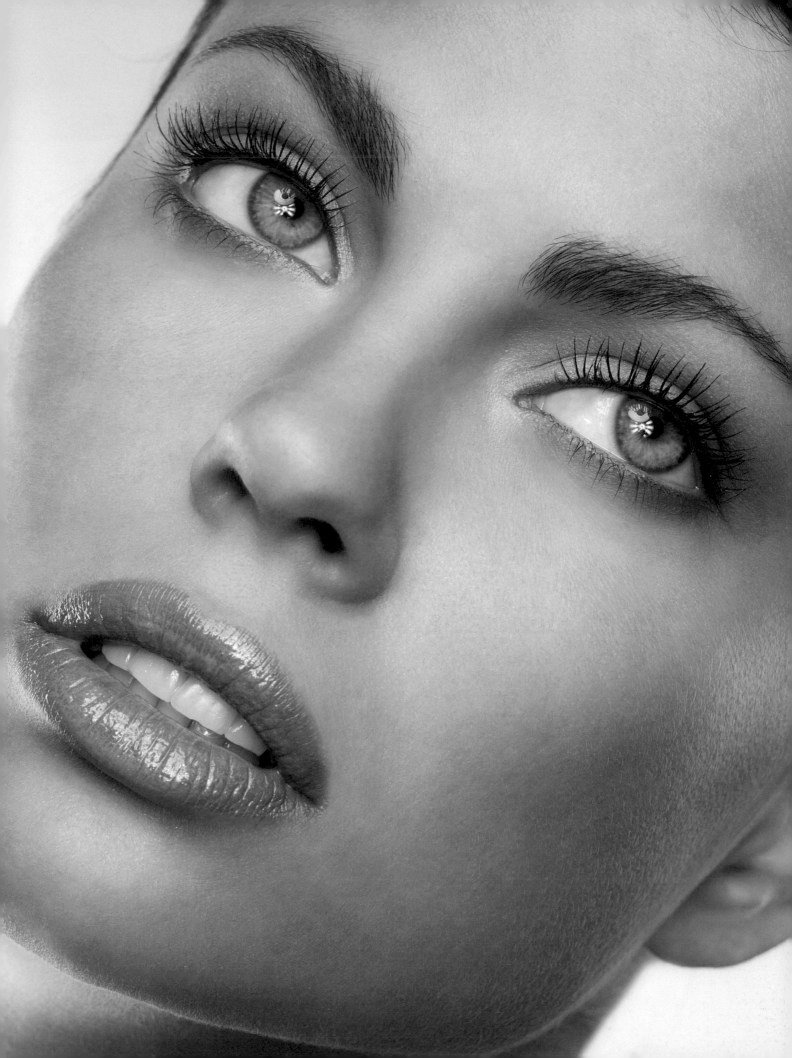

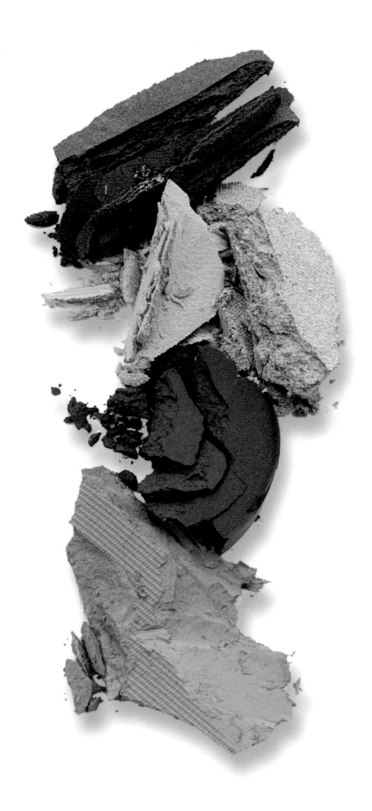

eyes

Your eyes always express your joy and happiness, especially on your wedding day. Because photography is an integral part of the day, it's important that your eye makeup accentuates rather than dominates your eyes.

Depending on the time of day and the lighting, your eyes can photograph very differently. I recommend staying away from really dark or unnatural eyeshadows, such as blue, green or black, and instead applying more natural shades of eyeshadows such as ivory, taupe, beige, or brown to bring out the color and sparkle in your eyes. Just make sure to always choose shades that enhance your eye color.

I recommend using three different shades of eyeshadow to achieve the most beautiful effect. Visit chapter 5, starting on page 77, for great application ideas and options.

To help your eyeshadow last longer, apply concealer and loose powder on your eyelids before applying your shadow. This will help absorb any excess oils and help your eyeshadows blend better. You can also first apply an eye primer, which is designed to keep the oils in your eyelids from mixing with the eyeshadow. You'll still want to follow the primer with concealer and loose powder to help the eyeshadow blend, because primer can hinder the blendability of your eyeshadow. By prepping your lid like this, everything will go on and blend beautifully.

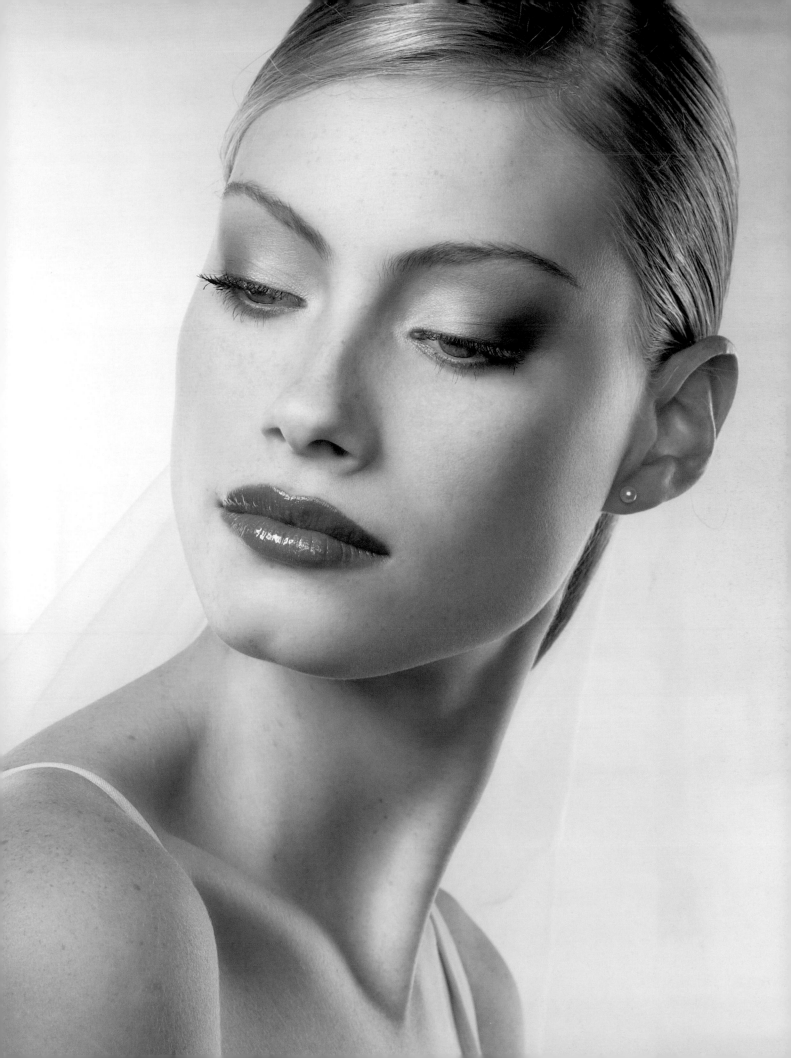

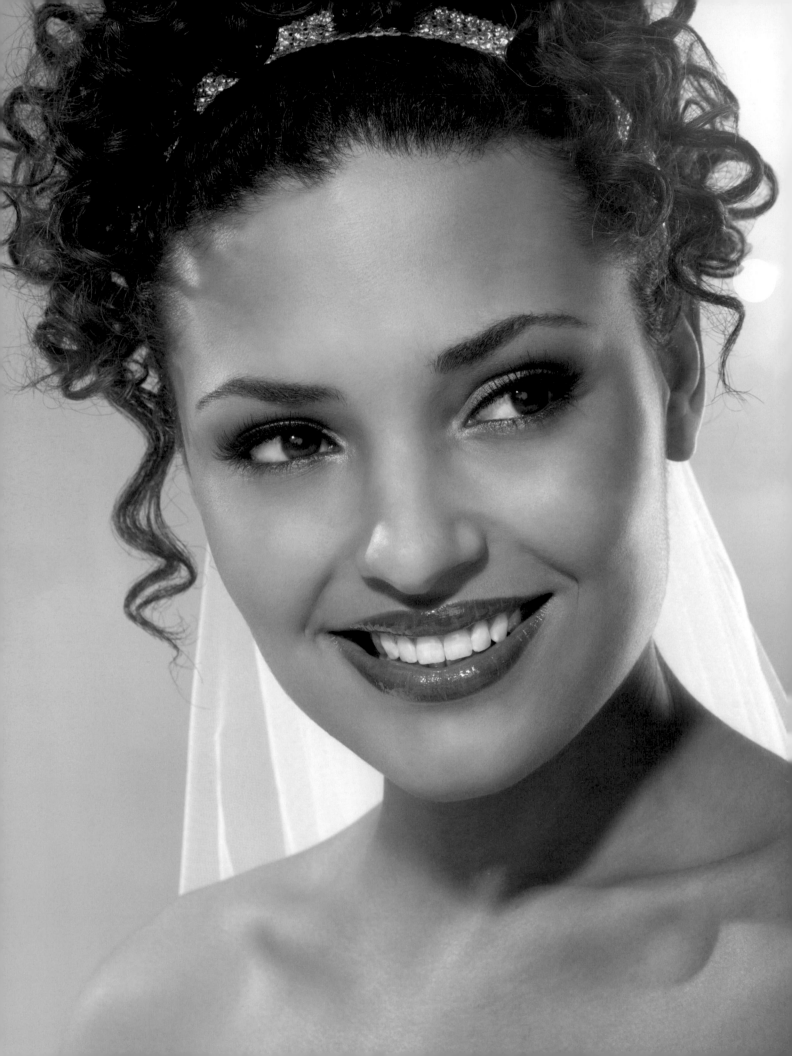

EYELINER

You can line and define your eyes in a number of ways: with pencil, liquid, cake, crème, or powder. Or you can skip this step completely! It's a matter of personal choice. Some women are under the impression that liner will always make their eyes look smaller, but that's not true if it's applied correctly. Well-applied eyeliner will actually open up your eyes and make them look bigger!

Pencil eyeliners are the most commonly used. Most now contain a bit of silicone, which helps it glide on and blend. For correct application, always make sure that the line along the top lashline starting at the inside of the lid is the thinnest, then gradually gets thicker as it extends to the outer corner. Along the bottom lashline, you want the color to be the most intense at the outer corner, slowly fading as it reaches the inner corner. Drawing the same thickness and intensity all the way across the top and underneath the eyelids can close in the eyes, and that's what makes them appear smaller. But applying it as I have just described will prevent that from happening. Many times, I don't even use pencil along the bottom lashline. Instead, I like to use an eyeshadow and a brush to create a softer, more natural look.

For perfect application, make sure you sharpen your pencil first. The sharper the point, the more precise the application. Now begin at the outside corner of your eye and draw small, featherlike strokes, connecting each one as you move toward the inside of the eye. Then blend with an eyeliner brush. Using the same eyeliner brush, apply a powder shadow in a similar color over the pencil to help make it look more natural. I always do this because it softens the pencil line and sets the color. It also helps you correct any mistakes you may have made when blending the pencil strokes together.

Liquid eyeliner is the longest wearing, and most brands come with a fine-tipped application brush. Liquid liner creates the strongest, most dramatic line. Never use liquid liner under the eye, because it leaves an unnatural line that can be stark and harsh in appearance.

When using liquid eyeliner on the top of your eyelid, draw a continuous line starting at the inside corner to the outside corner of the eye, giving the line a little "kick" upwards at the end. Make sure it is the narrowest at the inside corner, gradually getting thicker as you get to the outside corner. Liquid eyeliner is the most difficult to apply, but you can master it with a little practice. A helpful tip: Layer pencil and powder, then apply your liquid eyeliner. This is a trick that professionals use all the time to create a perfect line. Turn to page 80 to learn this professional technique.

Cake eyeliner comes as a powder. To apply, first dampen your eyeliner brush, then swipe it across the powder to form a liquid. Then apply it just as you would liquid eyeliner.

Crème eyeliner is also applied with a damp eyeliner brush in the same manner as liquid and cake.

Powder eyeliner, or eyeshadow used as liner, gives the most natural look and is the easiest to work with. You can use it dry or use it wet if you want a stronger look. To apply it dry, use an eyeliner brush and draw a fine line along the base of the lashes from the inside to the outside corner of the eye. If you would like to apply the powder wet, dampen your brush and apply it like liquid eyeliner. Powder used wet gives the same effect as liquid, but is much easier to control.

One of my favorite techniques is to take black eyeshadow and carefully push it into the base of the lashes (where the lashes grow out of the lid) using a small, shorthaired, flat-tipped brush. This defines the eyes and makes the lashes look thicker without making your eyes appear lined. It can really make your eye "pop."

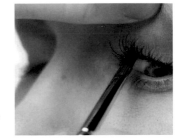

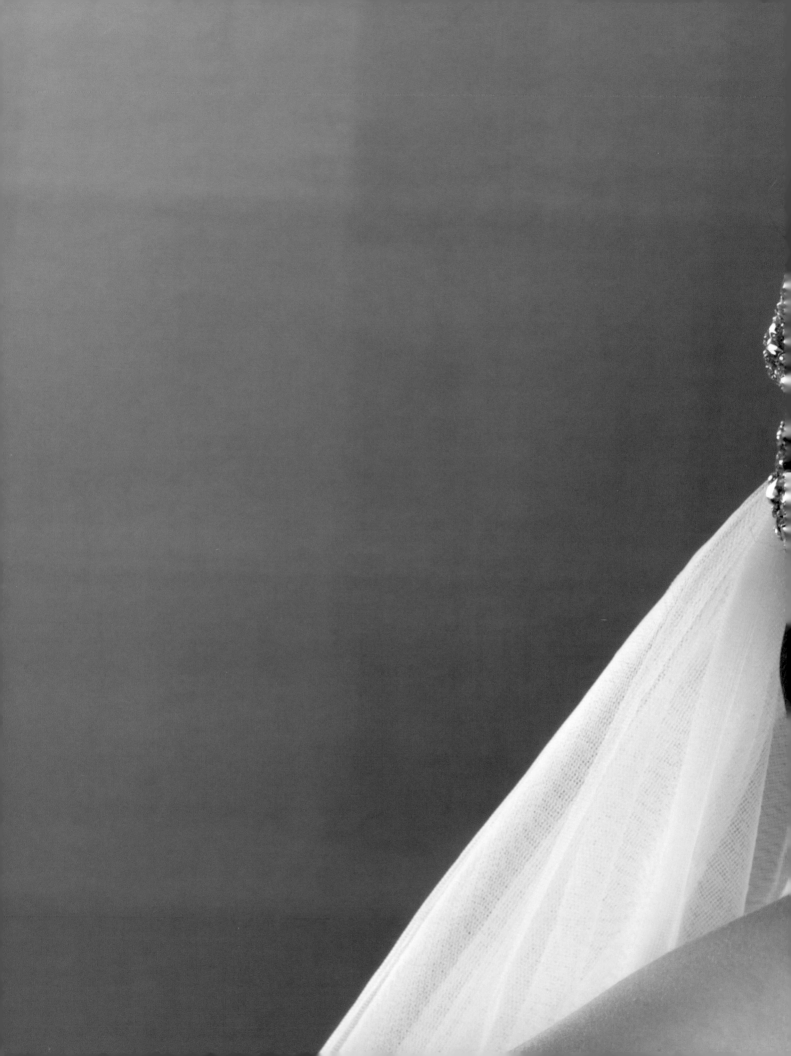

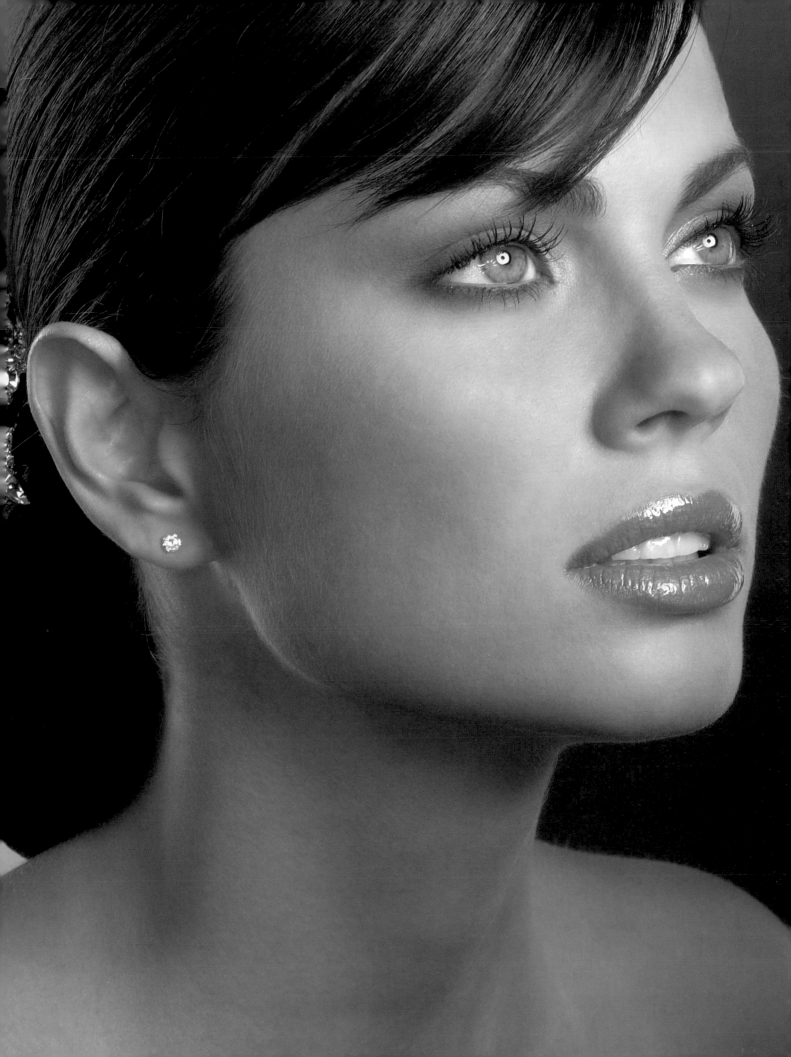

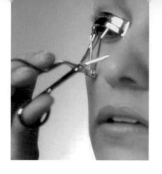
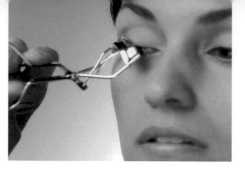
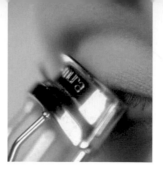
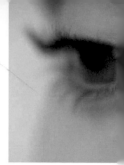

lashes

Fabulous lashes are always one of the best ways to define your eyes and make them stand out. Here are some great ways to get model-gorgeous lashes.

CURLING

I always recommend curling your eyelashes, because it opens up the eyes and makes them appear larger and more youthful. Many women skip this step, and it's a huge mistake.

The trick to curling your eyelashes correctly is not to crimp them more than once at the lash line. Instead, "walk" the eyelash curler up the length of your lashes, taking care to close, open, and move the eyelash curler up several times until you reach the end of your lashes. This method creates a curve rather than a crimp and will help your eyelashes stay curled. You should only use a crimp-style eyelash curler before you apply your mascara, never after. If used after, it could pull out eyelashes!

Thankfully, there is now an alternative eyelash-curling tool for those who are afraid of crimp-style eyelash curlers. You now have the option of using a heated eyelash curler. This tool is used after you've applied mascara. This is a great feature, as many times when you apply your mascara it can slightly uncurl your lashes. You simply push up and in with the curler, and your lashes will be curled to perfection —no crimping needed!

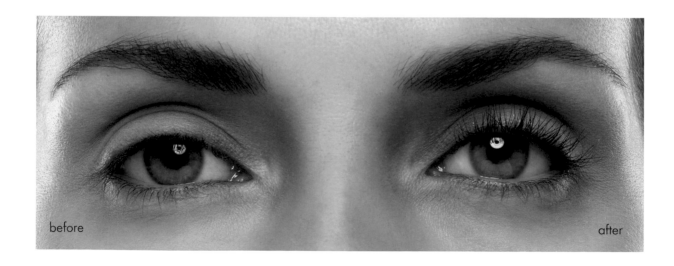

before

after

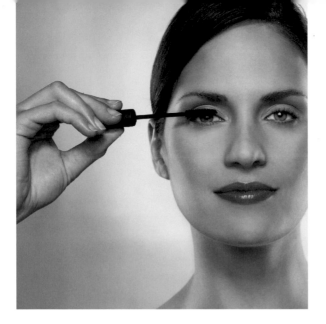
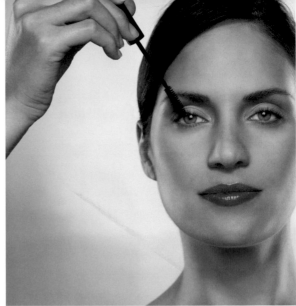

MASCARA

Mascara is everyone's favorite way to add definition to the eyes. I recommend applying several coats of mascara to define and open your eyes, since layering your mascara will give you the most dramatic definition. If you are concerned about getting teary-eyed during the ceremony or reception, make sure you finish with a coat of waterproof mascara.

Here's the best way to apply several coats of mascara to "build" lashes that last:

1. Curl your eyelashes with a crimp-style eyelash curler. (If you opt to use a heated curler, do so once you've applied your mascara and it's thoroughly dried.)

2. Pull the mascara wand out of the tube and wipe the brush against the opening of the tube to remove any excess product.

3. Apply the small amount that is left on the brush to your eyelashes.

4. Let each coat of mascara dry between each application. This could take a couple of minutes, so be patient.

   The trick to mastering multiple-coat application is making sure to apply very thin coats, letting each dry completely.

It's important to choose the correct formula of mascara for your desired effect. If you want to just define your eyelashes, use a defining formula. If you want to thicken and lengthen your lashes, choose a formula that will build.

Every girl wants long, thick lashes, and you can make your lashes look longer and/or thicker by applying your mascara correctly. Thickening and lengthening mascaras contain particles that attach to the lash to add bulk and length. But ultimately, you'll control whether or not your lashes appear longer and thicker by the application technique you choose.

For thicker lashes: Start at the base of the lashes and hold your mascara wand in a horizontal position, moving the wand from side to side as you work your way up to the end of the lashes. This makes the mascara particles attach to the sides of your lashes, making them appear thicker.

For longer lashes: Hold your mascara wand in a vertical position. Starting at the base of the lash line, pull the wand up and out to the end of your lashes. The particles will attach to the ends of your lashes, making them appear longer.

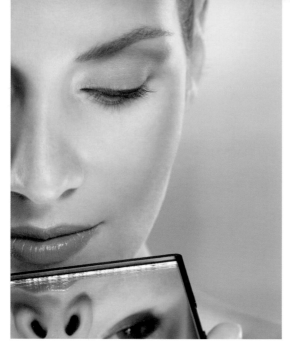

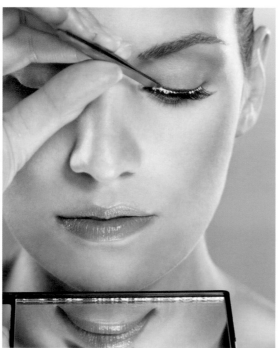

FALSE EYELASHES

Your wedding day is definitely the time to define your eyes. If you really want to draw attention to your eyes, you can always wear false eyelashes. I like using false eyelashes to define the eyes at the lashline instead of depending on heavy eyeliner and overly intense eyeshadow.

I know applying false eyelashes can seem intimidating, so here is an easy, foolproof way to apply false eyelashes. No matter what your makeup IQ is, this application technique will work for you and look natural. Just follow these easy steps to false eyelash perfection:

1. Curl your natural eyelashes.

2. Lay a mirror on the table or counter in front of you and look down.

3. Draw a thin line across your upper eyelid— right along your lashline—with an eyeliner pencil. This helps you know where to place the lash and helps conceal the lash band. This way, even if you do not get the false lash in place directly against your natural lashes, no one will know, because the liner will assure that no skin shows between your lashes and the false ones.

4. Trim the outside end of your false eyelashes to fit the width of your eyelid.

5. Apply eyelash glue to the false eyelashes. Allow the glue to dry for a minute so that it will get tacky (slightly sticky), then place the lash right on top of the eyeliner.

6. Once the glue has dried, apply one coat of mascara to blend your natural lashes with the false ones.

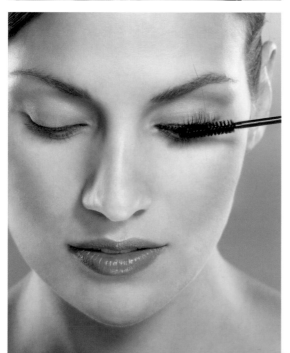

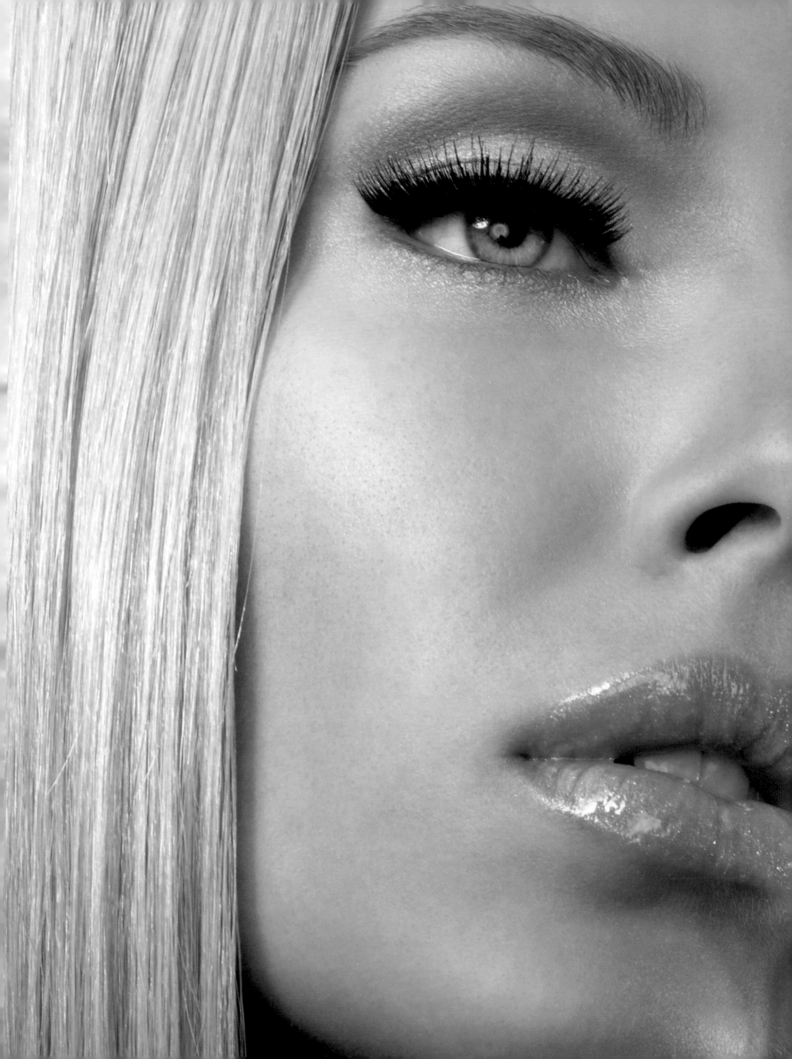

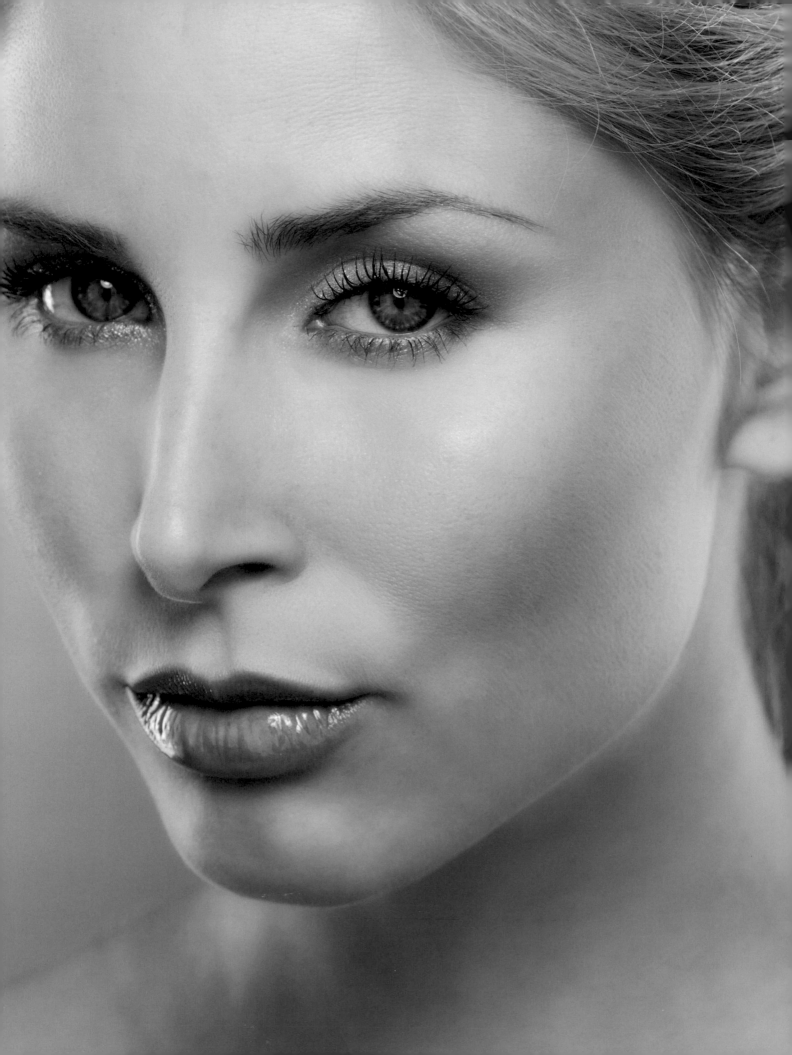

cheeks

Bronzer and blush work together to bring your face alive and give you a natural, healthy glow. Getting that beautiful glow is a two-step process, because I always like to bronze the face before adding the actual cheek color. I think every woman can benefit from bronzing, as it adds warmth and natural beauty to the skin and can make you appear younger.

Many women are confused as to where bronzer and blush should go on the face. I'm here to tell you that they belong on your cheekbones. If you know how to locate your cheekbones correctly, you'll always have your bronzer and blush in the right place.

To accurately locate your cheekbones, take this can't-miss application test:

1. Smile.

2. Locate the center of the "apple" of your cheek and place your index finger there.

3. Next, place your thumb at the top of your ear where it connects to your head.

4. Now take your thumb and bring it toward your index finger. The bone you feel is your cheekbone.

5. Next, apply your color directly onto the cheekbone.

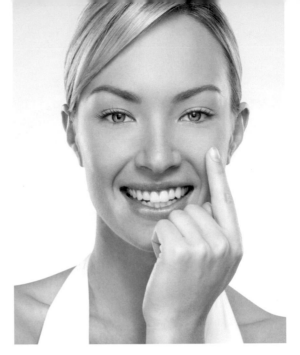

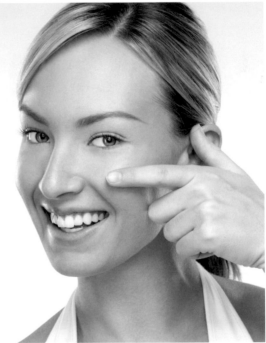

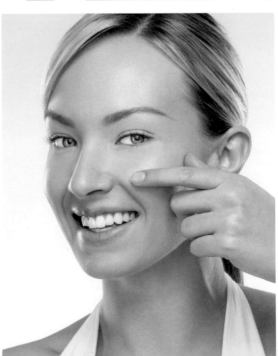

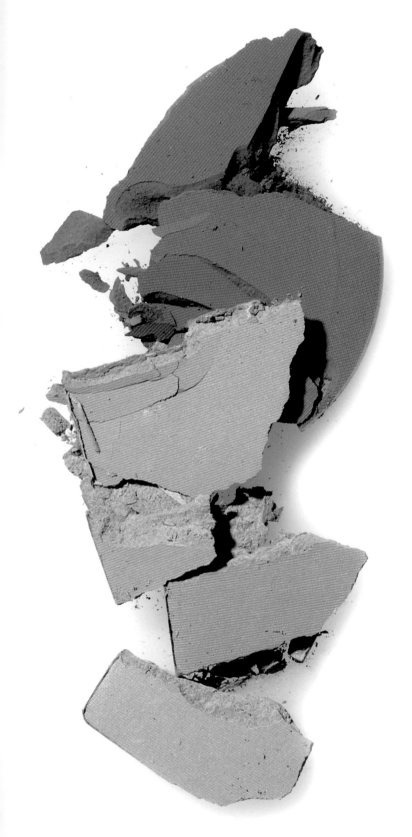

BRONZER

Bronzer makes your skin look sun-kissed and alive. It gives your skin a healthy glow without subjecting it to damaging ultraviolet rays. To warm your face and accentuate your bone structure, simply dust bronzing powder or crème bronzer along the outer edges of your face and onto your cheekbones. Bronzer is also useful for lightly "sculpting" the nose and chin. See page 90 for more on how to sculpt your face using bronzer.

Always apply your bronzer beginning at the back of your cheekbone, sweeping the brush forward toward the apple of your cheek then back toward your ear. This lays your color in place. Then take you brush and use it in the opposite direction (up and down) to blend. If you are using a crème bronzer, simply dot the color along your cheekbone and blend. Don't forget to add a little at the temples to help shape your face. Sweeping the bronzing powder up around the temples and eye sockets can also really help your eye color pop, especially if your eyes are green or blue.

If bronzing powders and crèmes look too bold on you, try using pressed powder instead. It has a lower pigment level and blends very nicely. If you have lighter skin, an ebony pressed powder will work beautifully as a bronzer.

BLUSH

The intensity of color you are wearing on your eyes and lips can determine the amount of blush you need that day. For example, if you are wearing a strong lip color, you will need less blush. If you are wearing a paler, sheerer lip color, you might need more blush.

Powder blush

A powder blush is the easiest to use. There are two ways to apply your powder blush properly:

1. Apply your blush along your cheekbone, starting at the back (closest to your ear). Sweep your cheek color toward the apple of your cheek, then back toward the ear again. Now go back again in the opposite direction (up and down) to blend. This way, your most intense color lies at the back of your cheek and gives your face more dimension.

2. For a more natural appearance, you can try a technique called "popping your apples." First, apply bronzer along your cheekbone, starting at the back. Sweep the bronzer toward the apple of your cheek, then back toward the ear. Now go back in the opposite direction to blend. Next, take a light, sheer blush color, making sure it is not too dark. Smile and apply your blush color starting at your apples and blending back toward the area that you bronzed. This gives the apples of your cheeks a beautiful glow. Again, you'll want to use a sheer shade of blush for this technique. A dark or bright cheek color can be too intense and unnatural looking.

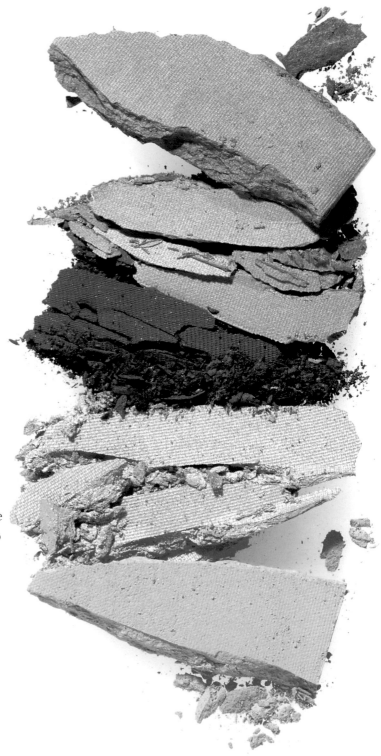

Crème or Liquid blush

If you use crème or liquid blush, apply it after your foundation and before your powder, and use either a sponge or your fingers for easier blending. If you wear your blush without foundation, crème and liquid work better than powder blush, because they contain moisture that blends better with the natural moisture of your skin. To apply crème or liquid blush, first dot a little onto the apples of your cheeks, and then blend back toward your ears.

BLUSHING BRIDE

Want to be a rosy-cheeked, blushing bride? One of the most important things to think about, as I have already mentioned, is making sure your color lasts. Here's an easy way to layer your cheek color and make it last from the ceremony to the reception, photo after photo:

1. After applying your foundation, apply a crème blush to the apples of your cheeks and cheekbones.

2. Dust your face with loose or pressed powder.

3. Apply a powder blush (similar in color to the crème blush) to the apples of your cheeks and cheekbones.

Using this application method will give you a bit more intense color, and everything will last throughout the evening. Don't forget to bronze your cheeks: It will keep your skin looking warm and glowing throughout your entire wedding day. You will just have to bronze after you apply your blush with this application technique, because you need to apply your crème after your foundation and before you powder.

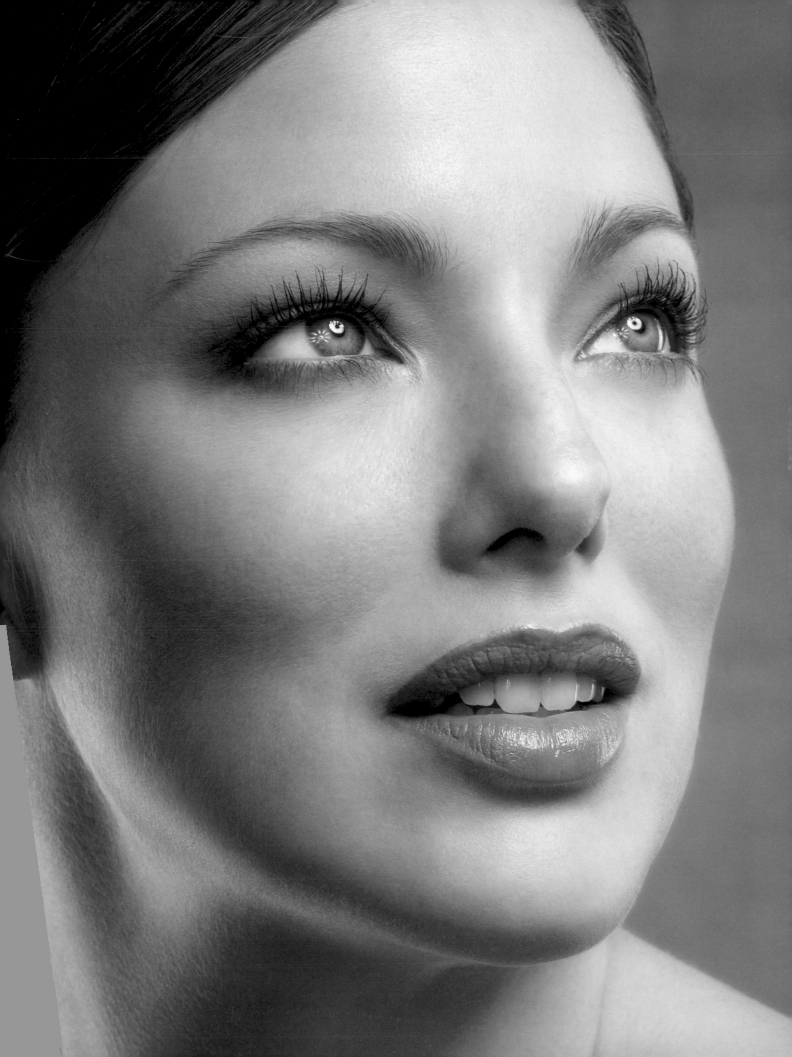

lips

To keep your lips looking luscious, exfoliate them once a week. To exfoliate, simply apply a generous layer of lip balm to your lips, let it soak in for a few minutes, then take a soft baby's toothbrush and brush your lips. You could rub them with a nubby-textured washcloth if you do not have a toothbrush handy. The balm will soften the dry skin so that when you brush your lips, you will remove the dry layer of skin, leaving your lips soft and smooth.

I always like to use a little lip balm or moisturizer on the lips before I apply lipstick color, because it helps the lip liner and lipstick go on smoothly and more evenly. Just apply the lip balm when you first start applying your makeup, at the same time you apply your moisturizer. This will give the balm time to soak in. Then, right before you apply your lip color, blot off the excess so the balm won't shorten your lip color's wearing time.

Lip pencil will help prevent lipstick from feathering and bleeding, but once you've outlined your lips, don't stop there. Be sure to blend inward, so that when your lipstick wears off, you aren't left with just an outline. You'll find a lip brush will help give you a more precise application and help everything blend better.

Make sure you optimize your entire mouth. Most women don't, because they tend to draw inside their natural lip line. Many times your lip line actually extends farther than the colored portion of the lip. Conversely, take care not to overdraw, because if you're using a lip color that is not natural-looking and you stray too far outside the lip line, it will be noticeable.

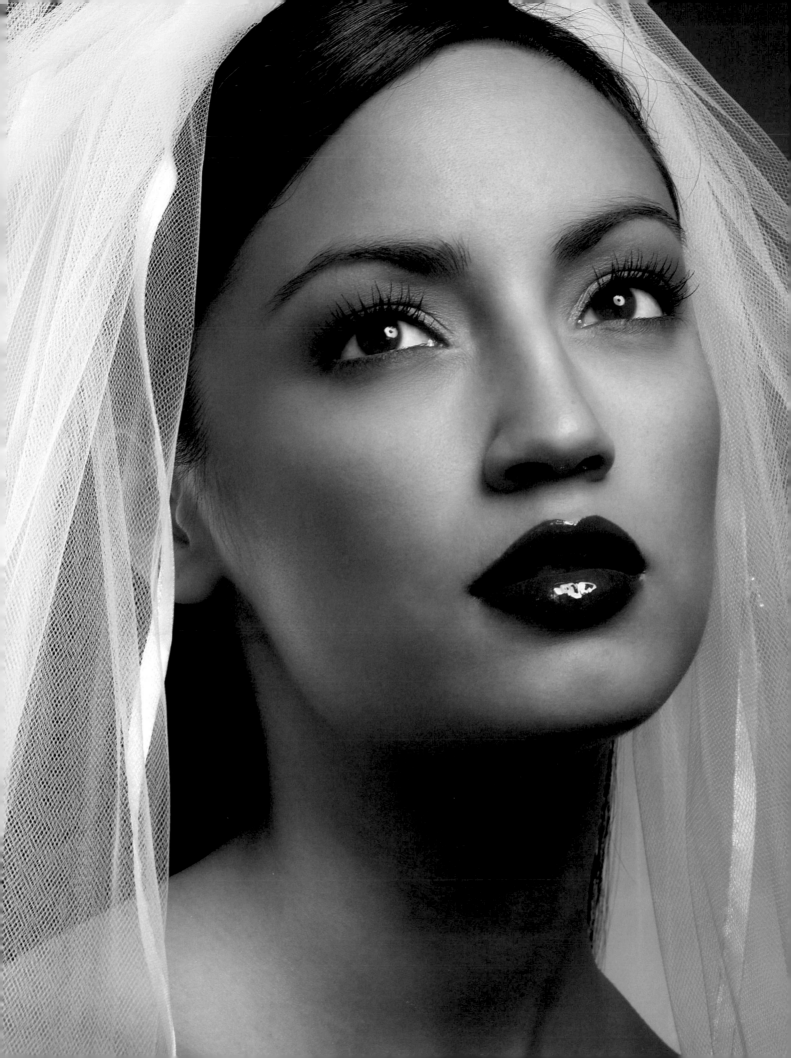

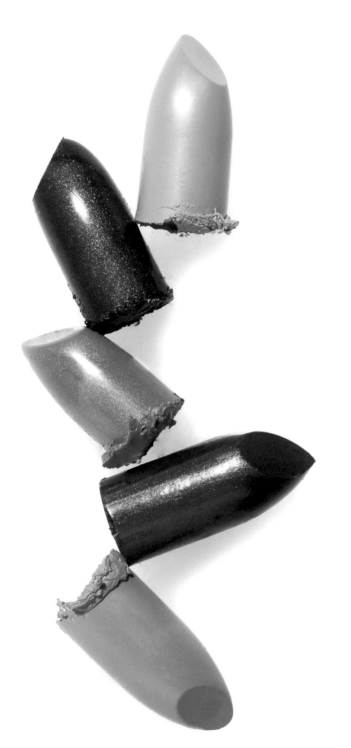

APPLICATION

To properly apply your lip liner to the top lip, begin with a V in the "cupid's bow" or center curve of the lips. Then starting at the outer corners, draw small, feathery strokes to meet the center V.

On the lower lip, first accentuate the lower curve of the lip, then begin small featherlike strokes from the outer corners, moving toward the center. Next, you can actually apply your color. You can use a brush, your fingers, or a tube to apply your lipstick, but if it's applied with a brush, it will usually look much more precise and last longer. For more intense color, you can apply it straight from the tube, but it will be harder to cover the smaller detailed areas of the lips.

LIP COLOR THAT LASTS

Since it is your wedding day, you want to give your lip color "stay-ability" so your smile looks beautiful all day. You do *not* want to constantly be touching up your lips. This is a good time to buy two of your favorite lipstick and lip gloss —one set to keep in your makeup bag, and one to stash in the groom's pocket for quick lip fixes and instant pretty smiles.

There are many ways to get your lip color to last. I have tried them all, and I have found in the end that there is one that really works best:

1. Conceal the entire lip area, everything from the natural lip line to the actual lip. This will create a more perfect edge for photos by hiding any discoloration you might have just outside your lip line, as well as creating the perfect canvas on which to apply your lip color.

2. Line the outer edges of the lips with lip liner, then fill in the entire lip area with liner. This is the first line of defense in getting your lip color to last. Lip liner has a drier texture than lipstick, so it lasts longer.

3. Next, apply a soft, pretty lipstick that looks natural yet still defines the lips. Then, take a tissue and gently blot your lips. This will remove the moisture from this layer yet leave you with a deposit of pigment. Next, reapply your lipstick; this time, do not blot. Layering color like this will give you double the pigment deposit, thus increasing how long the color will last.

4. Finish with a dot of lip gloss in the center of the lips to attract light and highlight your smile for photographs. I have found that lips with a bit of shine to them photograph more beautifully because the shine gives them dimension in a photo.

5. If you only want to wear lip gloss, make sure to line your lips and fill in the entire lip with pencil before applying the gloss. This will help your lip gloss last longer.

One great quick tip: If you have a groom who is concerned about ending up wearing your lipstick after the kiss, lick your lips before you kiss him. This will prevent the color from transferring. If you are wearing lip gloss and do not want the color to transfer, have him lick his lips before he kisses you. Then none of the gloss will transfer, thus leaving his lips color-free.

I usually discourage brides from wearing a dark lip color on their wedding day. It doesn't photograph as well as softer, more natural shades. The only time I'm okay with a dark lip color is if the bride wears it daily and it is part of her everyday look. If you choose to wear a dark lip color, remember you must wear soft eye shades so the two features don't compete with each other.

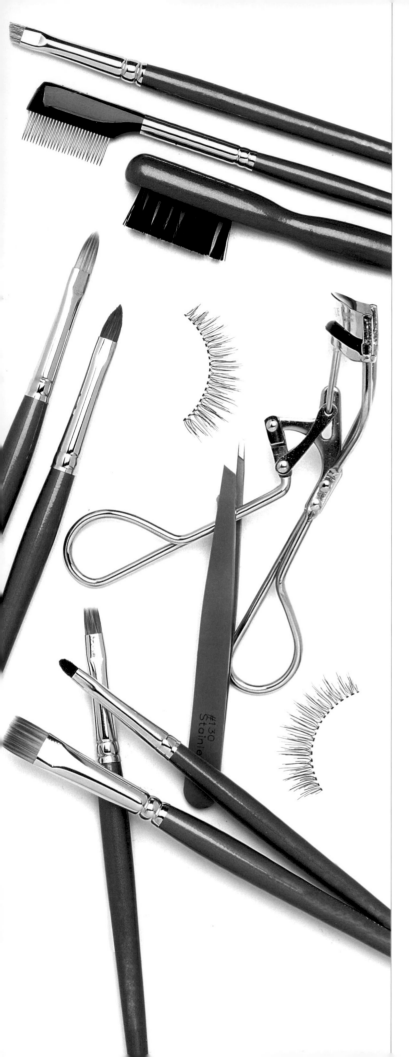

makeup must-haves

After you've decided on your look and favorite shades to wear, you'll want to pack your makeup bag with the beauty essentials on this list. The list contains everything you need to help you create a beautiful look and keep you looking radiant throughout your wedding day.

- moisturizer
- primer
- foundation
- concealer
- loose powder
- pressed powder
- bronzer
- brow color
- eyeliner
- eyelash curler
- mascara
- eye shadows
- false eyelashes (optional)
- blush
- lip pencil (2)
- lipstick (2)
- lip gloss (2)
- makeup brushes
- tweezers
- blotting papers
- sponges
- powder puff
- tissues

There are a few things on this list that I want to draw your attention to. Note that I've added the number "2" by a few of the products; you will need two of each of these products: one to put in your makeup bag for getting ready and one to use for touching up during the wedding.

Now I know most brides purchase a beautiful, expensive purse so you have a place to put your touchup makeup. But inevitably you gave the purse to Pam who gave to Tracey who gave it to Missy who gave it to Patty who can't remember where she put it, so when you need it, no one can find it.

I think the best place for those items is in the groom's jacket pocket. By the time you need them, you will be with him, and the darn purse is such a pain to keep up with anyway.

So the day before the wedding, give your groom your pressed powder, lip pencil, lipstick, lip gloss, and blotting papers to put in his pockets (he has at least three pockets). And if he is not willing to carry these small items for you, maybe you are marrying the wrong man!

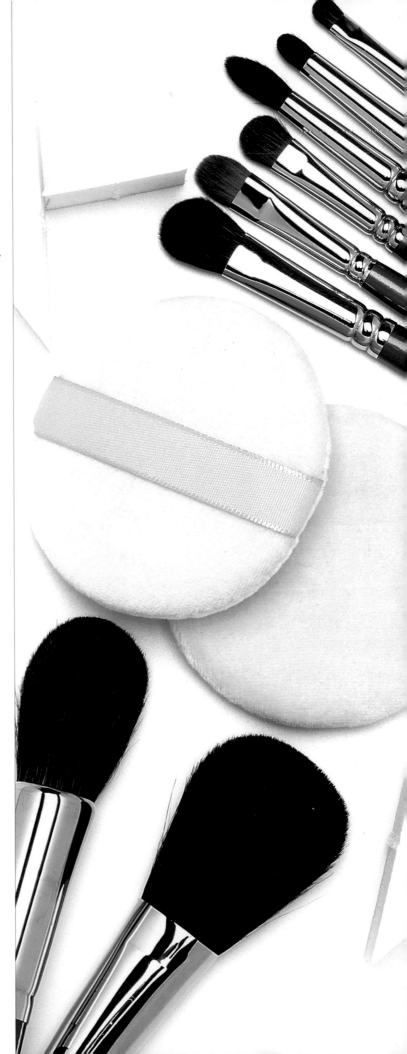

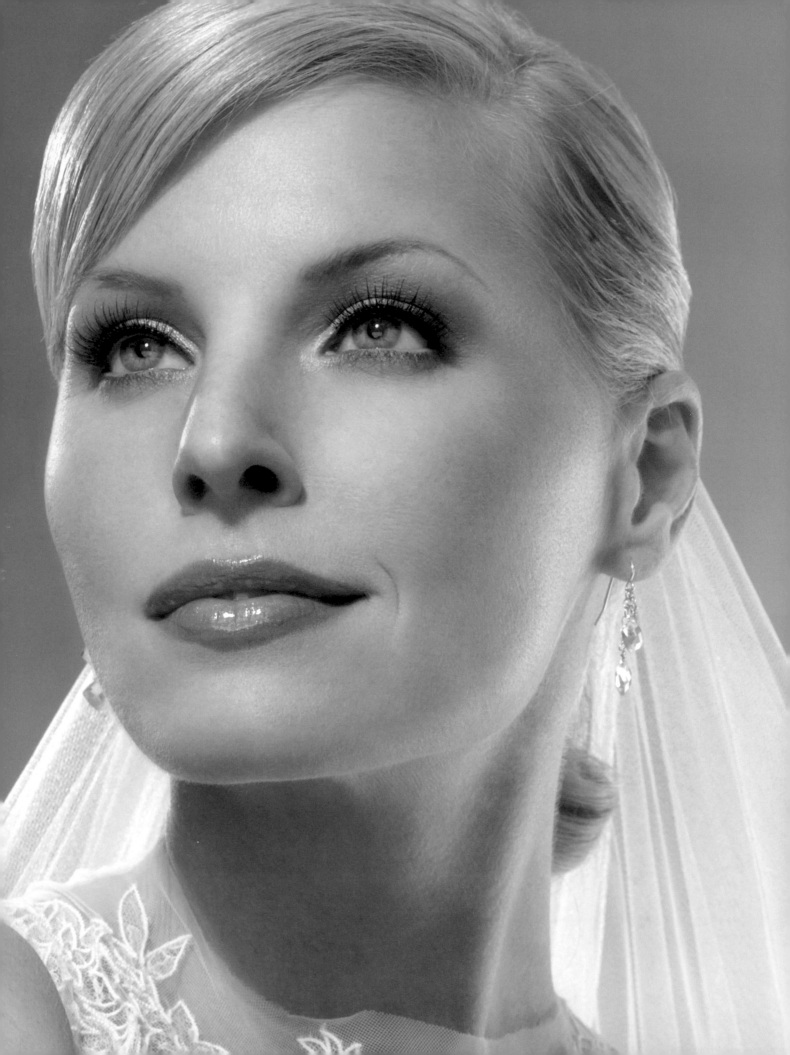

chapter five | create your look

This day is all about you and how beautiful you are, so I want to help you create the perfect makeup look for you. In my experience, the one most important feature to spotlight on your wedding day is your eyes. As they say, they are the windows to your soul. Well-defined, beautiful eyes always photograph fabulously! Here are some amazing makeup looks you can use to create the perfect eye look for you. I have also given you blush and lipstick suggestions to help complete each look. As always, experiment with these looks, and have fun long before your wedding day! You can try one or all, and choose the one you like best.

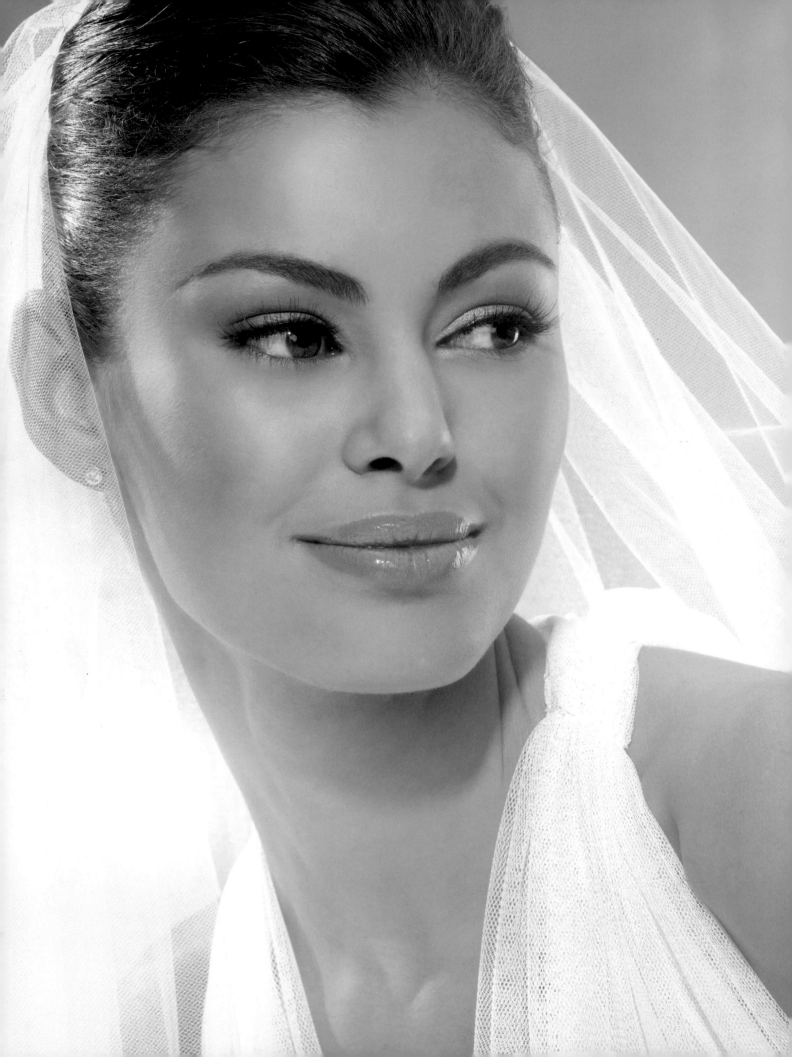

natural beauty

Eyeshadow is a great way to make the color of your eyes stand out and help define your eyes. If you simply want to bring out your natural beauty, this is a look that will be perfect for you. With this eyeshadow application, you can create everything from soft and natural to extremely dramatic, depending on your eyeshadow choices. To make sure you apply your shadows properly, follow the steps below for a simple application that will shape your eyelids and make you feel absolutely beautiful.

It takes three shades of eyeshadow to shape the eye: a highlight, midtone, and contour shade. Depending on the effect you want to achieve, your eyeshadow choices will make a big difference in the way you look. If you want to look soft and natural ,choose soft colors; if you want to look more dramatic, choose a contour shade that is deeper and richer in color.

APPLICATION:

1. Highlight shade: Apply to browbone, the lid, and inside corner of lower lashline.

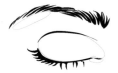 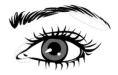

2. Midtone shade: Starting from the outside corner of the eyelid (because the first place you lay your brush gets the most color) gently move your brush across the crease into the inside corner of the eyelid. Also brush along the lower lashline, once again starting from the outside corner and brushing toward the inside, so that the most intense color is at the outside, fading as you move to the inside corner. This will help you create subtle definition.

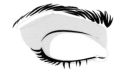 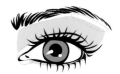

3. Contour shade: Apply across your upper lashline from the outside corner inward. Then bring the color up into the outer portion of the crease, and blend it inward about one third of the way, layering it on top of your midtone shade. Sweep color underneath the lower lashline for a soft, blended look.

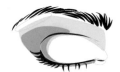 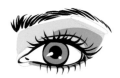

With this look, you have a multitude of blush and lip color options, depending on the intensity of eyeshadow you choose. For instance, if you choose a dark eyeshadow contour color, make sure you choose soft and subtle lip and blush colors. If you choose really soft and natural eyeshadow colors, you could choose a bit more intense lip and blush colors.

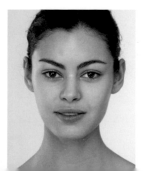

audrey hepburn eye

For a very sophisticated bride, this application technique will give you a simply beautiful look. This look is a modern take on the classic Audrey Hepburn look from *Breakfast at Tiffany's*. In the classic version of this look, there is no color along the bottom lashline. However, in our modern version, we are using your midtone eyeshadow shade to help create definition. This look is always beautiful and sophisticated.

APPLICATION:

1. Highlight shade: Apply to the browbone and the lid. Highlight the inside corner underneath the lower lashline (wrap the color around the inside corner of the eye) for added drama.

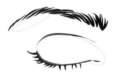 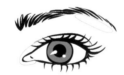

2. Midtone shade: Starting in the crease, apply your midtone color from the outer to the inner corner of the eye. Sweep the same color underneath the lower lashline for definition.

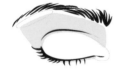 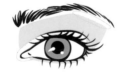

3. Eyeliner: Start by taking an eyeliner pencil and lining the upper eyelid first to start your pattern (perfect line). Start at the inside corner of the eye, and kick the liner upward at the outer corner. Make sure the line increases from thin to thick as you go toward the outer corner. Next, using a black shadow and an eyeliner brush, go over your pencil and fine-tune it, making it the perfect shape. Then follow the line with liquid eyeliner. Since you have first created the perfect pattern and then applied your liquid liner on top, if it is not perfect, no one will know, because you created the perfect shape first with your pencil and powder.

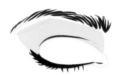 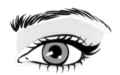

4. To really finish this look, apply false eyelashes. See page 62 for easy application steps.

When choosing a blush to go with this style of eye makeup, just remember that this is a classic look, so do not choose anything too strong or it could overpower your eyes. Unlike your blush, your lip choice could be a bit stronger with this eye look. Since it is soft and subtle, a little more intense lip color could look very sophisticated.

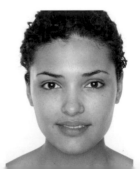

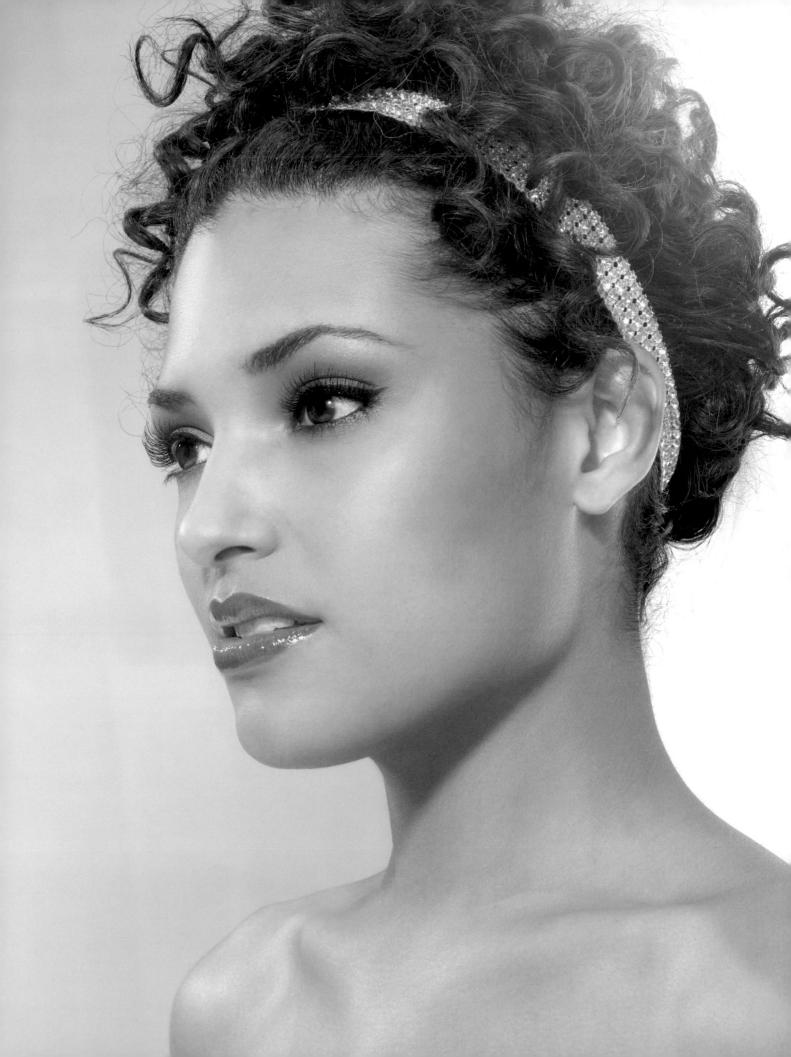

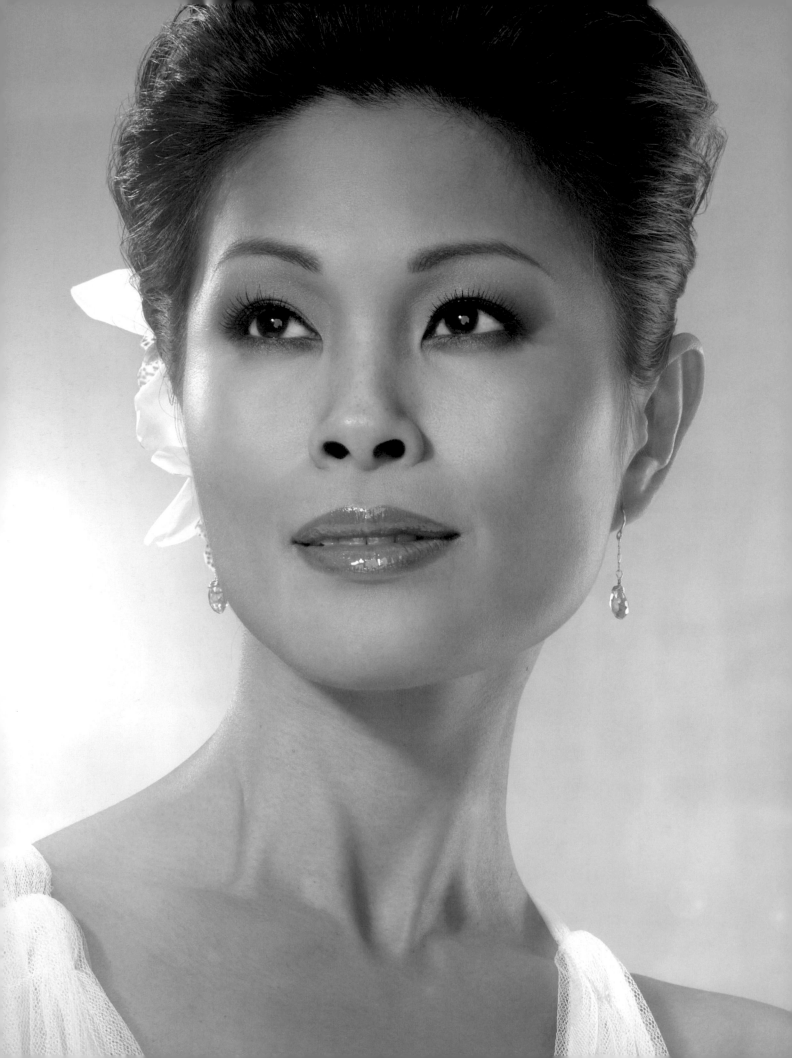

smoky eye

This look is perfect for the bride that wants a more dramatic look on her day. With this application technique, you will be able to create a sexy, smoky eye. Even though this is definitely a dramatic look, you control just how dramatic it is by choosing how dark your eyeshadow shades will be. You can use lighter shades and create a subtle effect, or choose darker shades for maximum drama. Whatever your eyeshadow color choice is, this application technique will define your eyes and make you look gorgeous in photographs.

APPLICATION:

1. Highlight shade: Apply to browbone only.

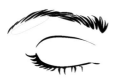 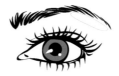

2. Midtone shade: Start at the base of your upper lashline, and bring the color up and over your entire lid—all the way up to your browbone. Also brush it along the lower lashline. This will help to create definition.

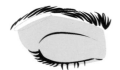 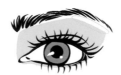

3. Contour shade: Again, start at the base of your lashline, and layer the color over your midtone all the way across your lid and up into the crease. Now sweep the contour color underneath the lower lashline as well. You'll create a light-to-dark effect with the three eyeshadows, with the darkest shade applied closest to the lashline and fading as you go toward the brow.

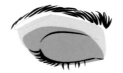 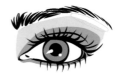

4. With this look, make sure you line your entire eye all along the top and bottom lashline.

With the smoky eye look, your eyes are the absolute focus. Soft, subtly glowing cheeks would look best. You can use color—just make sure it is a soft, sheer color so that it is not too intense for the eyes. If you choose deep, rich eyeshadow colors, make sure you wear a very soft, subtle lip color. You never want both your eyes and lips to be dark! Your lips should be as subtle as possible; close to nude would be best. It would look fantastic if you chose just to wear a really soft, beautiful lip gloss with this look. A soft gloss color would not be too strong and fight with your eyes for attention.

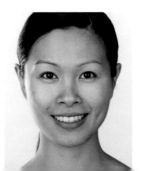

sparkling eye

Put a twinkle in your eye and give yourself a fresh glowing look. Nothing is more beautiful than a look with a bit of sparkle and shine to the eye. The key to this look is to create the shine or sparkle on only the eye. You want to make sure the rest of your face has very little shine to it. Your skin should be matte, your blush should have no shimmer to it, and your lips should not be too glossy. The only shade that should have shimmer to it is your highlight shadow.

APPLICATION:

1. Highlight shade: Apply a sparkly highlight shade to your browbone and lid. Make sure to highlight the "V" on the inside corner of the eye (wrap the color around the inside corner). This will really accentuate the shimmer and sparkle.

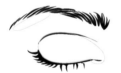 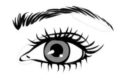

2. Midtone shade: Starting from the outside corner of the crease, sweep the color across to the inside corner of your eye. Also brush it along the lower lashline, once again starting from the outside corner and brushing toward the inside, so that the most intense color is at the outside, fading as you move to the inside corner. This will help you create subtle definition. Make sure this shade is matte.

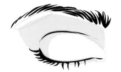 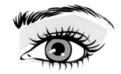

3. Contour shade: Sweep the color along the upper lashline and into the crease, layering it on top of your midtone shade. Apply underneath the eye all along the lower lashline. Make sure this shade is also matte.

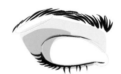 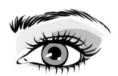

When making blush and lip choices, you want to make sure you don't overpower the sparkly eye that you have just created. Remember: no shimmer to your blush! Make sure you choose a soft, subtle shade that will give your cheeks a glow. You can wear a lip gloss if you like, but make sure that it will not overpower your eyes.

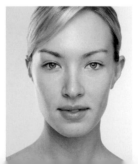

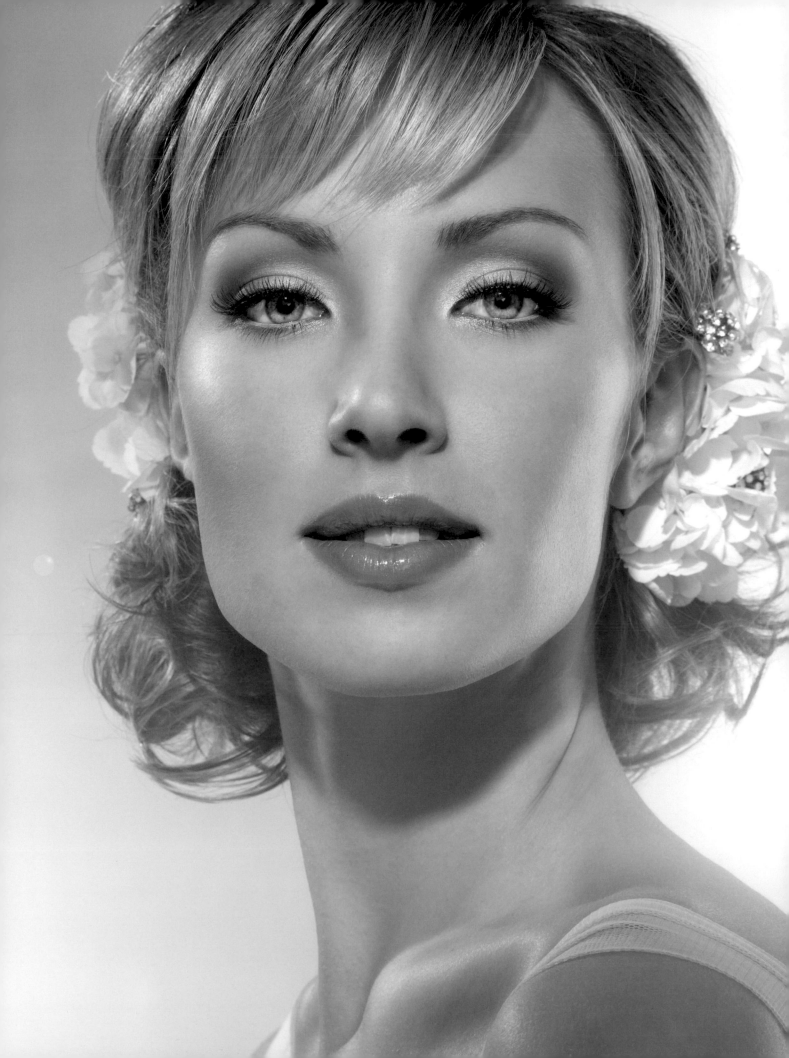

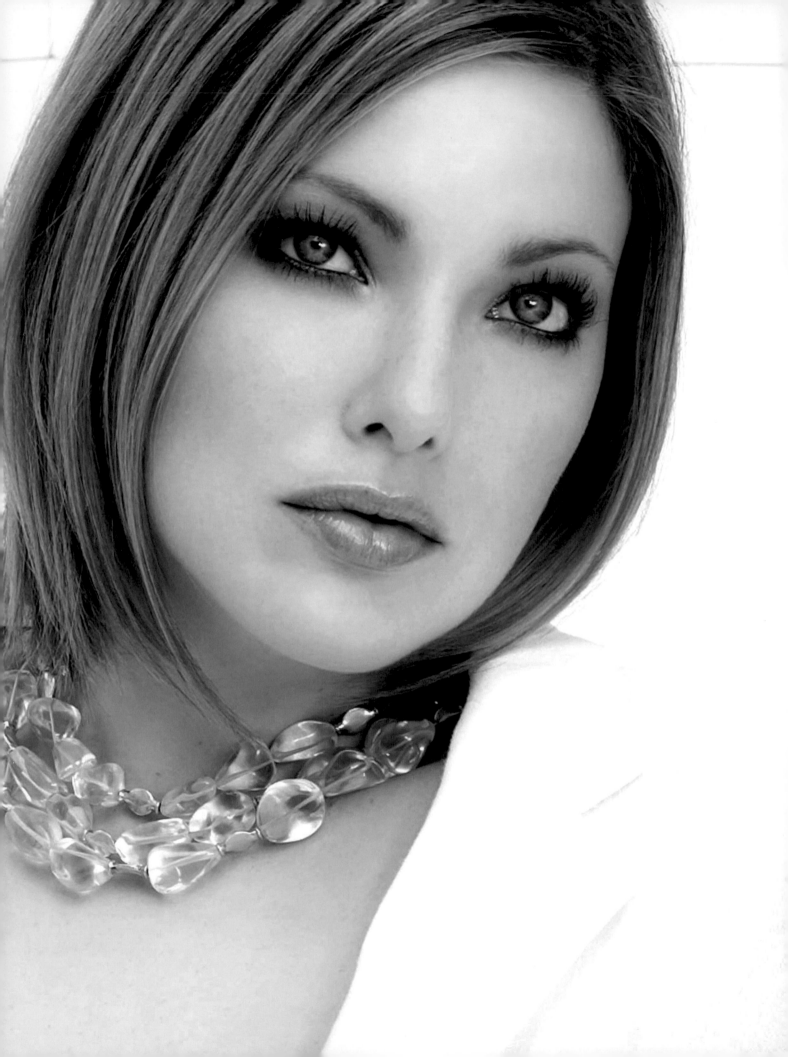

matte	nude	highlight		matte	ginger	midtone	
matte	sand	highlight		matte	mahogany	midtone	
shimmer	flesh	highlight		shimmer	pinkish brown	contour	
shimmer	beige	highlight		shimmer	purple	contour	
shimmer	gold	highlight		shimmer	chocolate	contour	
shimmer	coral	highlight		shimmer	golden brown	contour	
matte	taupe	midtone		shimmer	burgundy	contour	
matte	rose	midtone		matte	mahogany	contour	
matte	dark taupe	midtone		matte	dark brown	contour	
matte	caramel	midtone		matte	charcoal	contour	

I have put together a comprehensive chart of eyeshadow colors that I have used to create all the looks in this book. I've given you a palette with a wide array of colors, so every woman can find a look that she will love.

The names are generic, so you can compare with any cosmetic line and find these shades. Simply by using the chart on this page, you can see what specific eyeshadow shades I used to create all the bridal looks in chapter 7.

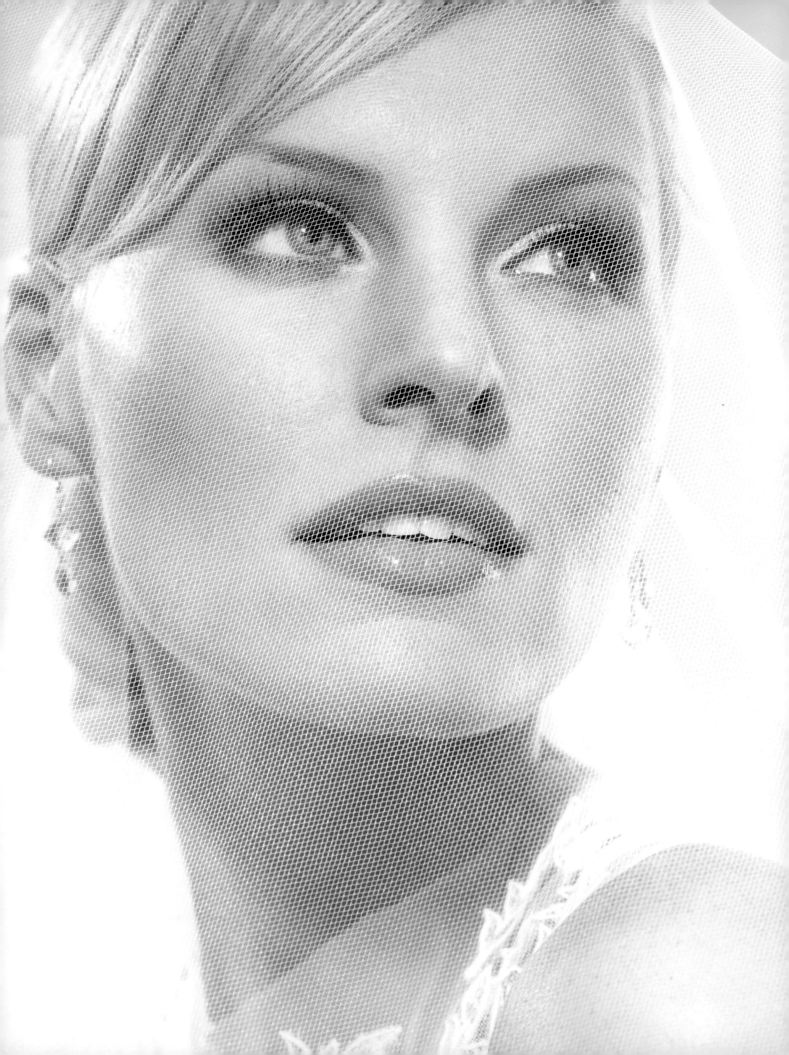

chapter six | picture perfect

In my opinion, the most important thing to think about when preparing for your wedding is how you will photograph. Many, many years from now, when the wedding dress no longer fits, the only tangible thing you will have to really remember your special day are the photographs.

So when considering your makeup look for your wedding photos or your bridal portrait, remember that it's all about making your best features stand out in the photo. You want to define your features better—not cover everything up with heavier makeup.

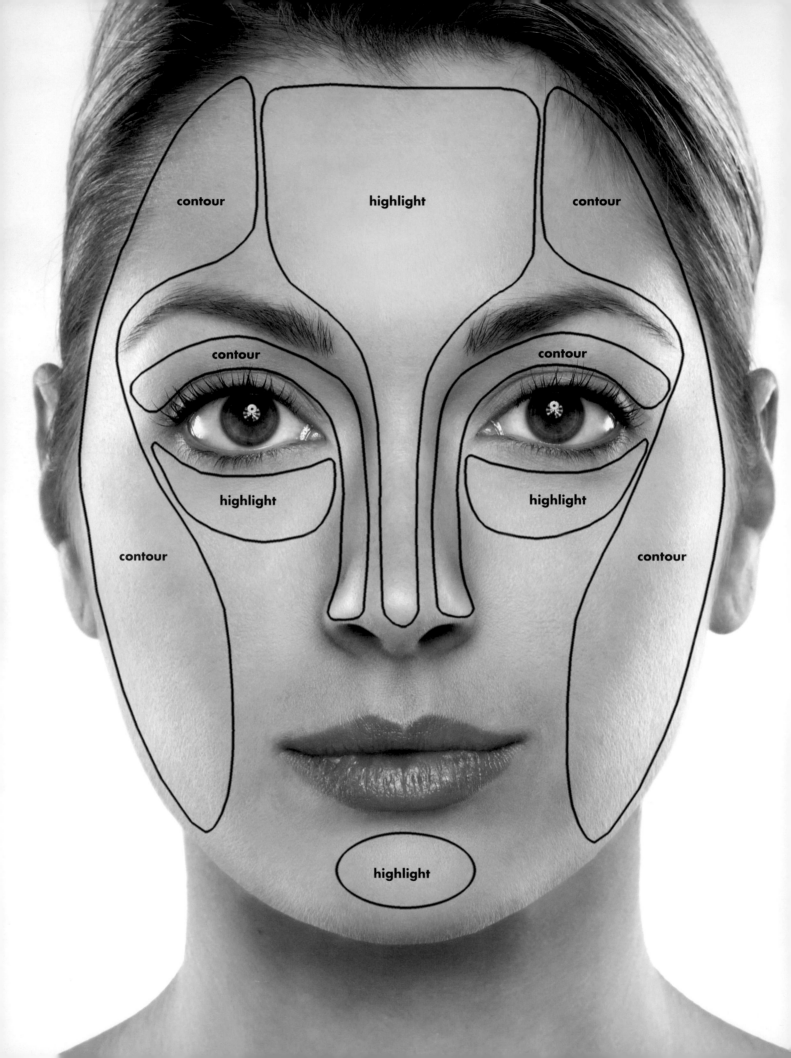

Depending on the lighting and the camera's flash, professional photography can wash you out and make you appear pale. But we can prevent that from happening. The best way to make your skin appear warm and radiant is to sculpt the face using highlighting and contouring techniques. This will give your face more dimension in your bridal portrait and help you photograph more beautifully.

You will need three shades of foundation to achieve this "face-sculpting" effect. The diagram on the left will help you understand the purpose and placement of the three shades. Be sure to blend the three shades really well, because it is the blending that makes the sculpting method work and look natural. Here's how it works:

1. The first color should match your skin exactly. It is your true foundation color. Apply this shade all over your face.

2. The second color—your highlight color— should be one level lighter than the first. Apply this shade to the high points of your face, including your forehead, under the eyes on top of the cheekbones, and on the tip of your chin. This helps to give your face more dimension by bringing these areas of the face forward.

3. The third shade—your contour color— should be one level darker than your first (natural) shade. Apply this shade to the outer areas of your face, including the temples, along your hairline, and along the sides of your cheeks. This will deepen your skin tone and help you appear healthier and warmer so you don't look washed

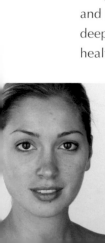

out. It also adds dimension and depth to your face while still looking very natural. To complete your look, you can simply finish with the shade of powder that matches your natural foundation shade.

This will still let your sculpting efforts shine through. But if you want to really enhance your sculpted look, follow what you have done with three shades of powder: one that matches your first foundation shade, one that matches your highlighter shade, and a darker or bronzing powder to match your contour shade. This will give you a perfectly sculpted face that will photograph beautifully.

Powder is the most important makeup step when doing photography makeup, because it eliminates shine and helps the skin appear smooth and matte—the perfect canvas for beautiful pictures. Matte skin always looks more perfect and flawless than shiny skin.

Here's an easy trick if you want to narrow the width of your nose: Create a strip of highlight shade down the center of your nose the width that you want your nose to appear. Then place the contour shade on the sides of your nose. This will make your nose look narrower, because the eye will be drawn to the highlighted area. If your nose is a little crooked, bring a straight line down on the top of your nose with the highlighter shade, then contour along the sides. People will naturally focus on the line that is highlighted, making the nose appear straight.

Blending is also key when it comes to professional photography makeup. The softer the light, the more perfect your makeup and skin need to be. The brighter the light, the less perfect your skin and makeup have to be. Bright light tends to "blow out the skin" and diminish the fine details. In softer light, the camera can pick up a makeup line along the jaw, neck, or eye area, so be sure to blend in your foundation, cheek, lip, and eye colors extremely well.

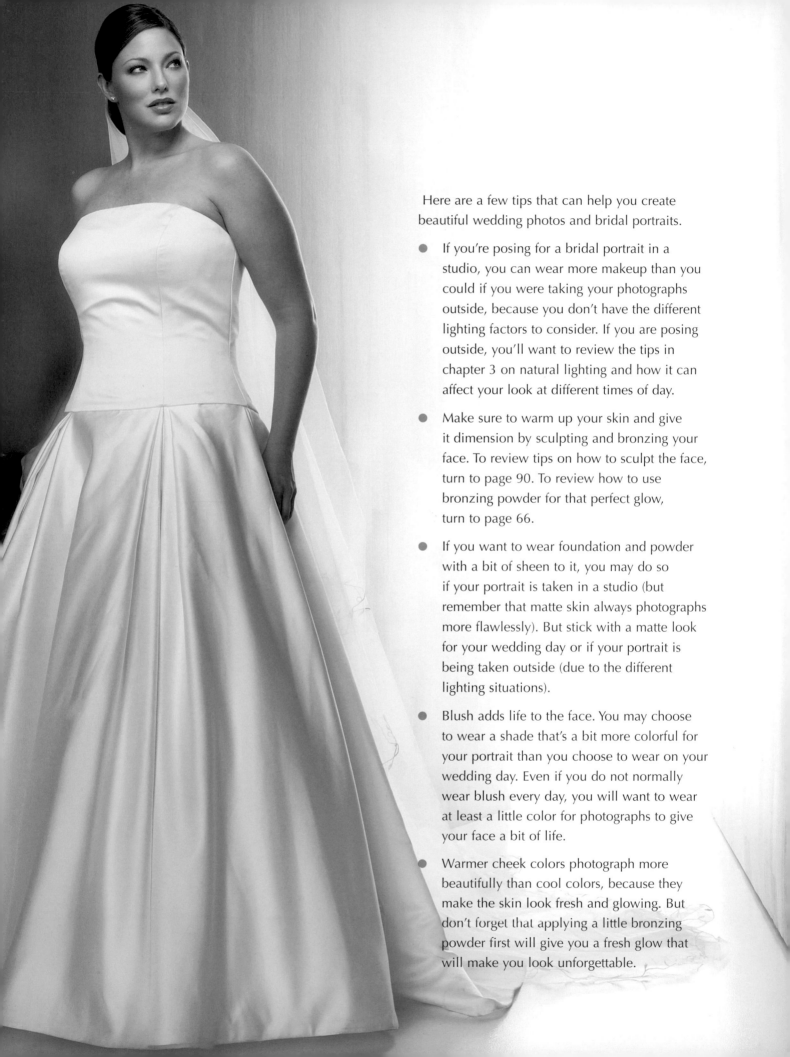

Here are a few tips that can help you create beautiful wedding photos and bridal portraits.

- If you're posing for a bridal portrait in a studio, you can wear more makeup than you could if you were taking your photographs outside, because you don't have the different lighting factors to consider. If you are posing outside, you'll want to review the tips in chapter 3 on natural lighting and how it can affect your look at different times of day.

- Make sure to warm up your skin and give it dimension by sculpting and bronzing your face. To review tips on how to sculpt the face, turn to page 90. To review how to use bronzing powder for that perfect glow, turn to page 66.

- If you want to wear foundation and powder with a bit of sheen to it, you may do so if your portrait is taken in a studio (but remember that matte skin always photographs more flawlessly). But stick with a matte look for your wedding day or if your portrait is being taken outside (due to the different lighting situations).

- Blush adds life to the face. You may choose to wear a shade that's a bit more colorful for your portrait than you choose to wear on your wedding day. Even if you do not normally wear blush every day, you will want to wear at least a little color for photographs to give your face a bit of life.

- Warmer cheek colors photograph more beautifully than cool colors, because they make the skin look fresh and glowing. But don't forget that applying a little bronzing powder first will give you a fresh glow that will make you look unforgettable.

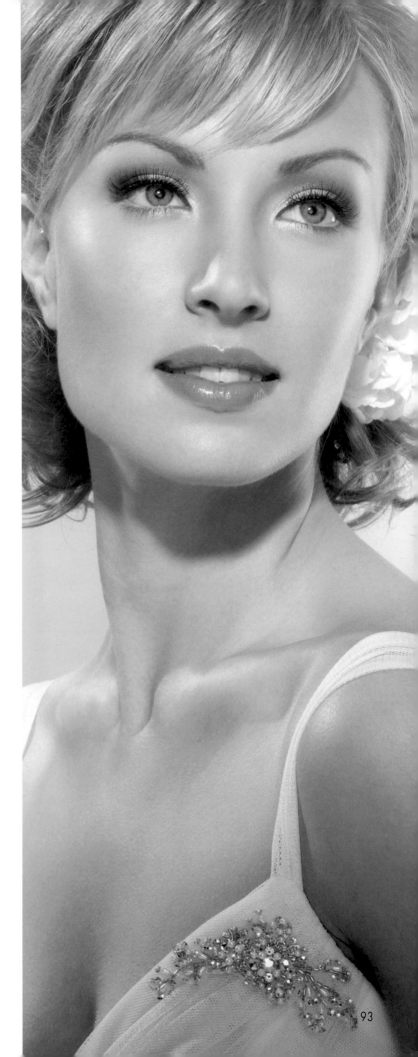

- You can wear matte or shimmer eyeshadows for your portrait and your wedding day but never frosted shadows. They always look too shiny and artificial in photographs. Remember, this picture is forever!

- Make sure at least one of your eyeshadows has a matte finish. Generally, you never want to use three shades of shadow with a shimmer because they will make the lid look too shiny. It is okay, however, to use three matte shades. For me, the one shade I almost always choose to be matte is my midtone, because it is supposed to look the most natural.

- When choosing eyeshadows for photography, shades with warm undertones (including brown) enhance every eye color and will photograph beautifully.

- Don't choose shades that are too bold. This is not the time for bright fuchsia lipstick or charcoal eyeshadow. Instead, you should choose lip shades that are just a few shades darker than your natural lip tone. Select eyeshadow shades that are deep enough to create definition and enhance your eye color, but not dark enough to demand all the attention. Your goal is to define your features with enough color to see the definition in the photographs, but not so much that you overwhelm and distort your features.

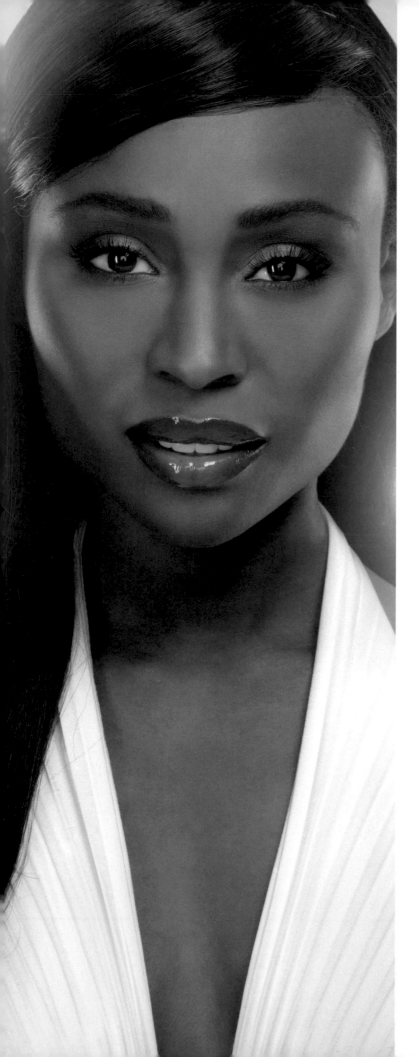

- Nothing will bring out your eyes better in a photograph than defining really well at the lashline. There are two ways to achieve this. First, you could layer your mascara to help thicken and lengthen your lashes. Turn to page 61 to learn how. The second technique—and my favorite for the absolute best definition—is to apply false eyelashes. Turn to page 62 for foolproof application tips.

- Make sure your lips are well defined for your portrait. Erasing your natural lip line with foundation or concealer before you apply your color will give you a fresh, perfect canvas, so that when you apply your lip liner it will give your lips perfect definition in photographs.

- Brows should be well groomed and defined with brow color. Even if you do not normally wear eyebrow color, in a photograph, the light could possibly wash your brows out, so a little color for definition might be necessary.

- I know I have already mentioned it, but I want to end by reminding you again that powder is your friend when you're being photographed. Matte skin always photographs more flawlessly than shiny skin!

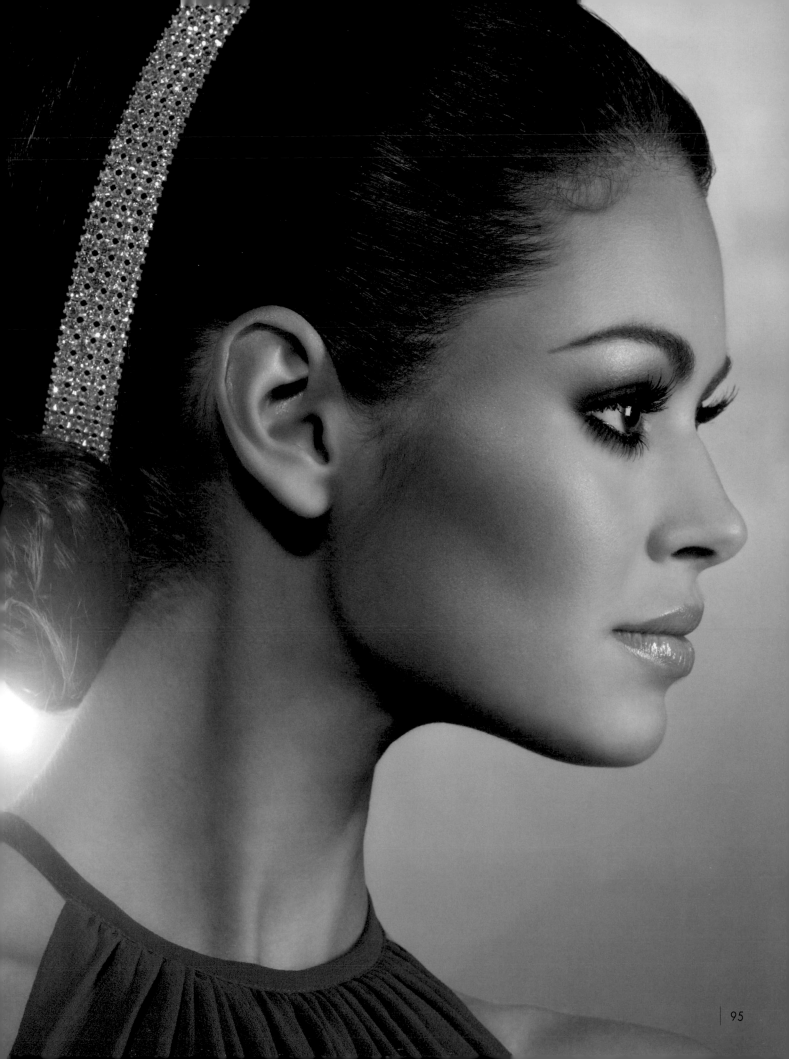

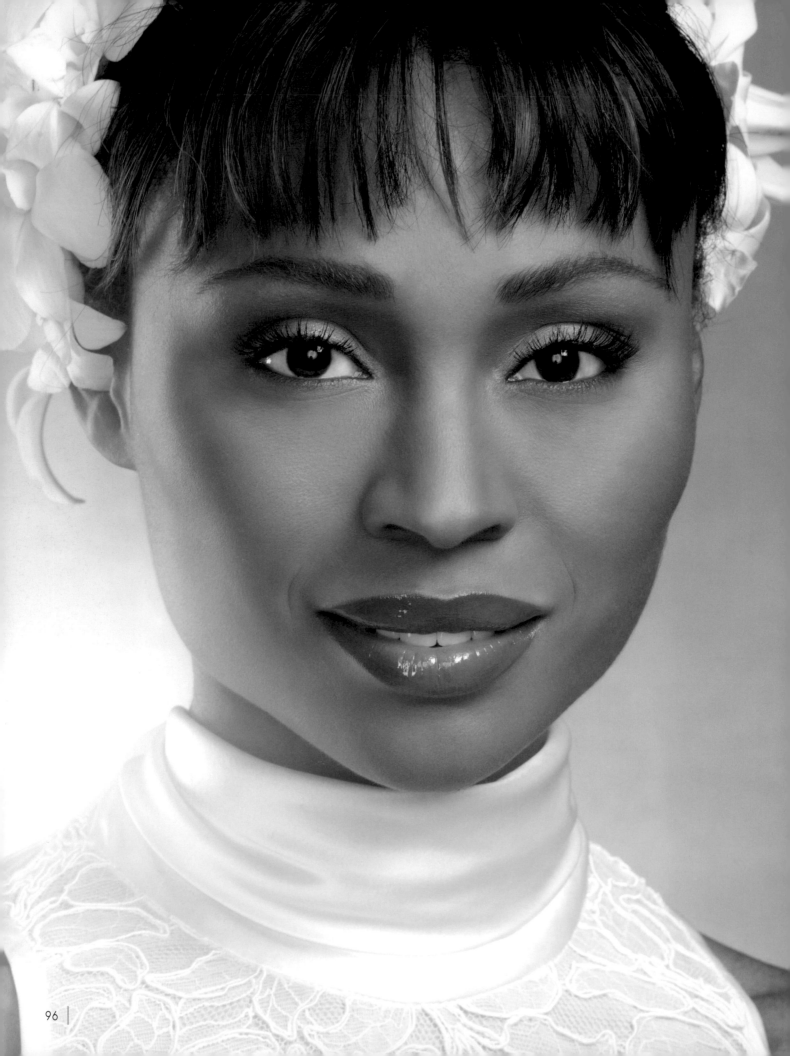

chapter seven | # bridal inspiration

In this chapter, I have gathered together some before and after photographs to show what makeup looks really work to make a beautiful bride. I have listed the eyeshadow applications I have used for each look as well as the time or times of day these looks will photograph most beautifully. I have also listed the blush and lipstick shades used. With all this information, you will surely be able to create the perfect look for you! Remember to try many different looks before your wedding, since you never know what you might discover.

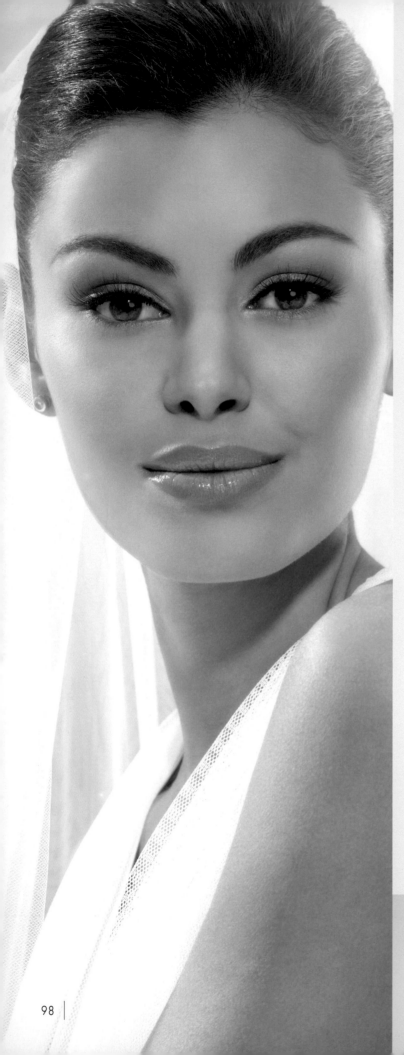

nonna

WEDDING TIME:	morning/midday/ late afternoon/evening
EYESHADOW APPLICATION:	natural beauty (page 79)
EYESHADOW:	highlight: shimmer beige midtone: matte taupe contour: shimmer pinkish brown
EYELINER:	taupe
BLUSH:	rich honey
LIP LINER:	flesh
LIPSTICK:	pinkish nude
LIP GLOSS:	creamy nude
TIPS:	This look works perfectly for any time of day, because it is so subtle yet it defines every feature. Notice how I really achieved a lot of definition on the eyes with thick, dark long lashes. Choosing subtle lip and blush colors gives the entire look a beautiful natural appeal.

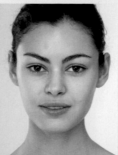

eleanor

WEDDING TIME:	late afternoon/evening
EYESHADOW APPLICATION:	smoky eye (page 83)
EYESHADOW:	highlight: shimmer gold midtone: matte caramel contour: shimmer burgundy
EYELINER:	rich brown
BLUSH:	rich honey
LIP LINER:	warm caramel
LIPSTICK:	soft peach
LIP GLOSS:	shimmer coral
TIPS:	Normally I would only let a bride wear a smoky eye during an evening wedding, but because I chose softer eyeshadow shades and still used a smoky eye application, she could also wear this look for a late afternoon wedding. Don't forget that a subtle lip shade will still be the best choice.

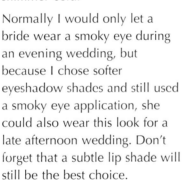

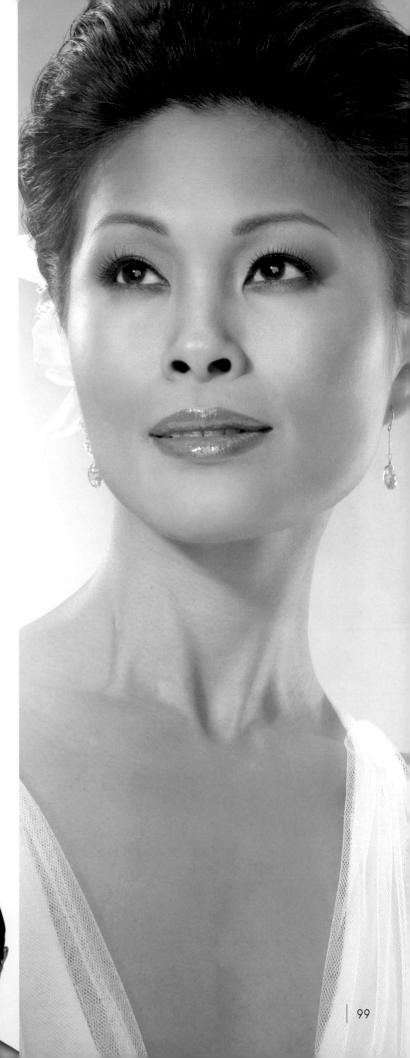

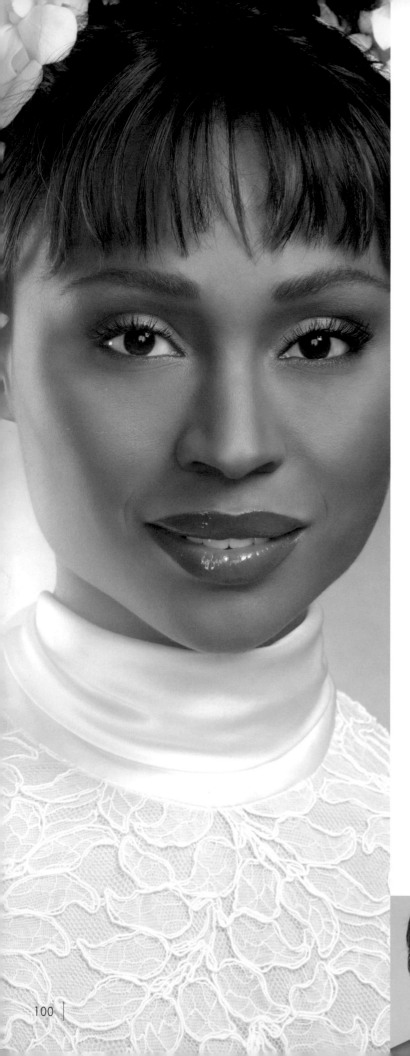

cynthia

WEDDING TIME:	morning/midday/ late afternoon/evening
EYESHADOW APPLICATION:	natural beauty (page 79)
EYESHADOW:	highlight: shimmer coral midtone: matte ginger contour: shimmer chocolate
EYELINER:	rich brown
BLUSH:	rich terracotta
LIP LINER:	warm caramel
LIPSTICK:	golden nude
LIP GLOSS:	shimmer bronze
TIPS:	Because this look is so natural yet defines every feature, it is perfect for any time of day. What makes it so versatile is the fact that my shade choices are subtle and natural but still add all the definition a bride needs, even for an evening wedding.

marisol

WEDDING TIME:	late afternoon/evening
EYESHADOW APPLICATION:	natural beauty (page 79)
EYESHADOW:	highlight: shimmer flesh midtone: matte taupe contour: matte dark taupe
EYELINER:	taupe
BLUSH:	rich honey
LIP LINER:	burgundy
LIPSTICK:	rich berry
LIP GLOSS:	shimmer berry
TIPS:	I would normally never do a dark lip for a wedding. But since it is a part of Marisol's everyday look, it is appropriate for her. I still kept in mind the time of day of the wedding, though. If it had been a morning or midday wedding, it would have been a "no go" on the dark lip!

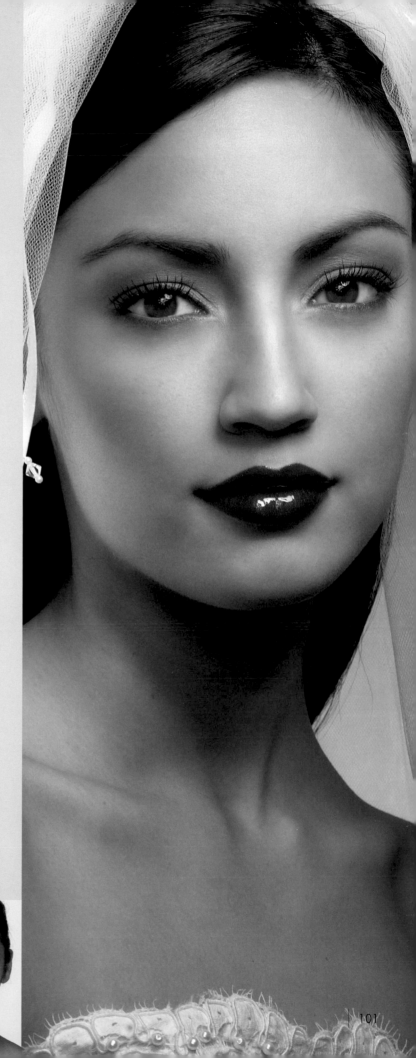

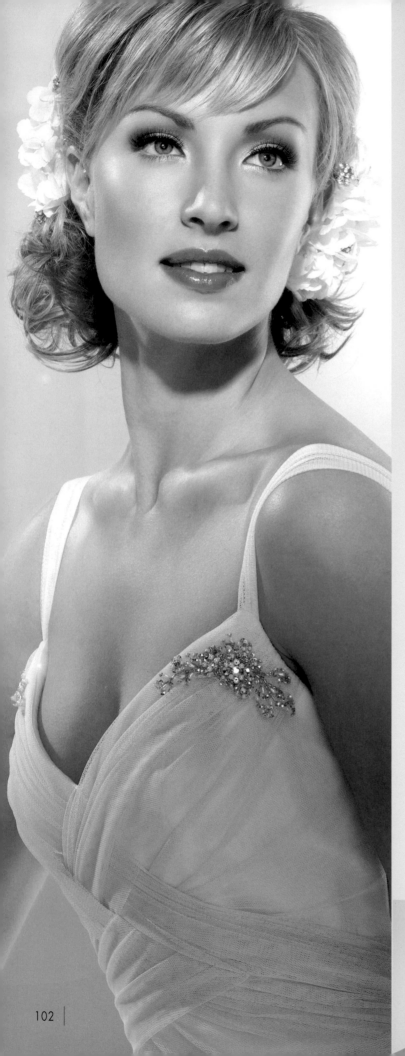

kate

WEDDING TIME:	midday/late afternoon/evening
EYESHADOW APPLICATION:	sparkling eye (page 84)
EYESHADOW:	highlight: matte nude/ shimmer flesh midtone: matte taupe contour: matte dark brown
EYELINER:	rich brown
BLUSH:	warm pink
LIP LINER:	flesh
LIPSTICK:	warm pink
LIP GLOSS:	creamy nude
TIPS:	To make the shimmer highlight eyeshadow shade show the most, I first layered a matte nude color on the lid (to create a base), then applied the shimmer highlight eyeshadow shade on top to make it stand out even more. Notice that I still concentrated on creating a really strong defining line at the lashline for the most intense definition.

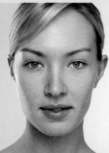

carol

WEDDING TIME:	morning/midday/ late afternoon/evening
EYESHADOW APPLICATION:	audrey hepburn eye (page 80)
EYESHADOW:	highlight: shimmer gold midtone: shimmer pinkish brown
EYELINER:	charcoal
BLUSH:	rich terracotta
LIP LINER:	warm caramel
LIPSTICK:	golden nude
LIP GLOSS:	shimmer berry
TIPS:	Carol's look works at any time of day because it is a classic. But I have taken that classic look and given it a modern twist. You can never go wrong with simply being beautiful!

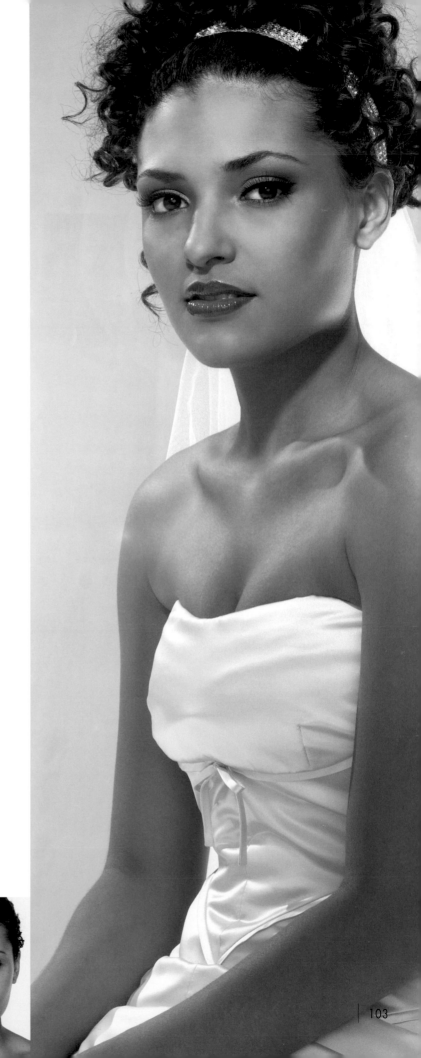

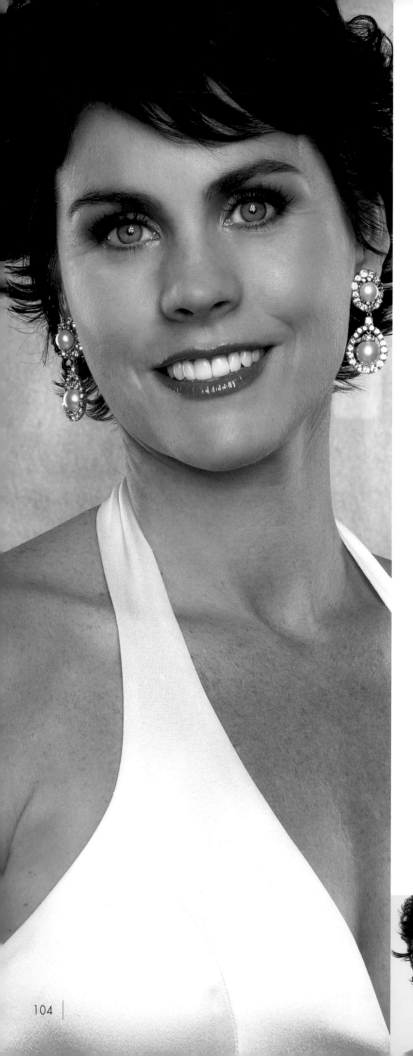

jamie

WEDDING TIME:	morning/midday/ late afternoon/evening
EYESHADOW APPLICATION:	natural beauty (page 79)
EYESHADOW:	highlight: shimmer beige midtone: matte taupe contour: shimmer golden brown
EYELINER:	bronze
BLUSH:	soft apricot
LIP LINER:	warm caramel
LIPSTICK:	warm pink
LIP GLOSS:	shimmer warm pink
TIPS:	Jamie's look is simple and natural, which is one reason it works at any time. I put the most intense eyeshadow colors at the base of the lashes. This will give Jamie's eyes the definition that I am looking for, but still keep her looking soft and natural.

gayle

WEDDING TIME:	late afternoon/evening
EYESHADOW APPLICATION:	sparkling eye (page 84)
EYESHADOW:	highlight: shimmer beige midtone: matte caramel contour: matte dark brown
EYELINER:	rich brown
BLUSH:	rich honey
LIP LINER:	warm caramel
LIPSTICK:	soft peach
LIP GLOSS:	shimmer coral
TIPS:	To make the shimmer highlight eyeshadow shade show the most, I first layered a matte nude color on the lid (to create a base), then applied the shimmer highlight eyeshadow shade on top to make it stand out even more. Normally, a sparkling eyeshadow application will work at any time of day, but because I chose eyeshadow shades that are a bit deeper, Gayle's look would be best for late afternoon or evening.

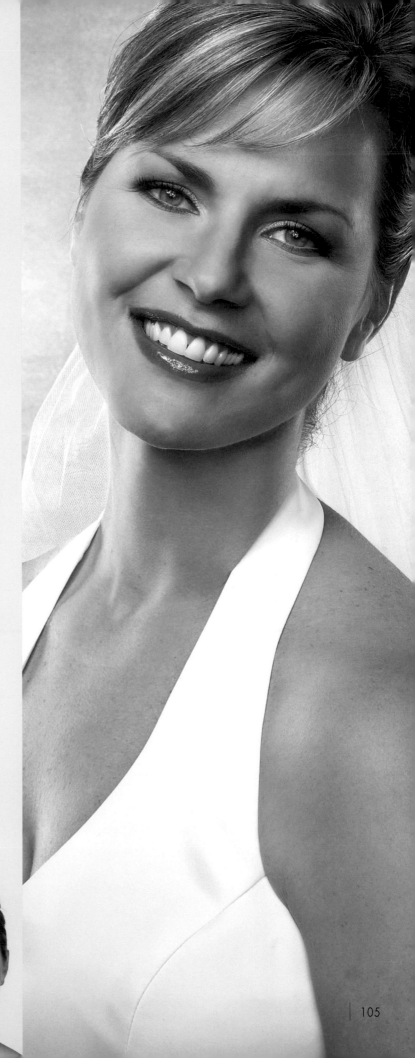

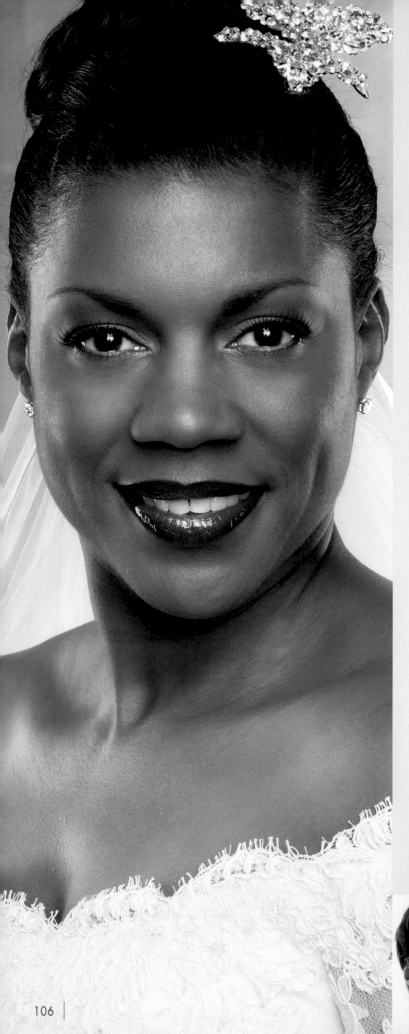

maxine

WEDDING TIME:	midday/late afternoon/evening
EYESHADOW APPLICATION:	natural beauty (page 79)
EYESHADOW:	highlight: shimmer gold midtone: matte mahogany contour: shimmer burgundy
EYELINER:	rich brown
BLUSH:	rich terracotta
LIP LINER:	burgundy
LIPSTICK:	rich berry
LIP GLOSS:	shimmer berry
TIPS:	For Maxine's look, I chose to make her lips the attention-getter, rather than her eyes. That is why I chose a bit darker and richer lip color and chose slightly softer eyeshadow colors.

missy

WEDDING TIME:	late afternoon/evening
EYESHADOW APPLICATION:	smoky eye (page 83)
EYESHADOW:	highlight: shimmer flesh midtone: matte taupe contour: matte mahogany
EYELINER:	rich brown
BLUSH:	soft peach
LIP LINER:	warm caramel
LIPSTICK:	soft peach
LIP GLOSS:	shimmer coral
TIPS:	Normally, I would only let a bride wear a smoky eye during an evening wedding, but because I chose softer eyeshadow shades and still used a smoky eye application, Missy could also wear this look for a late afternoon wedding. But don't forget that, even though we have used soft eyeshadow shades, we must still keep the lip soft so as not to overpower the bride!

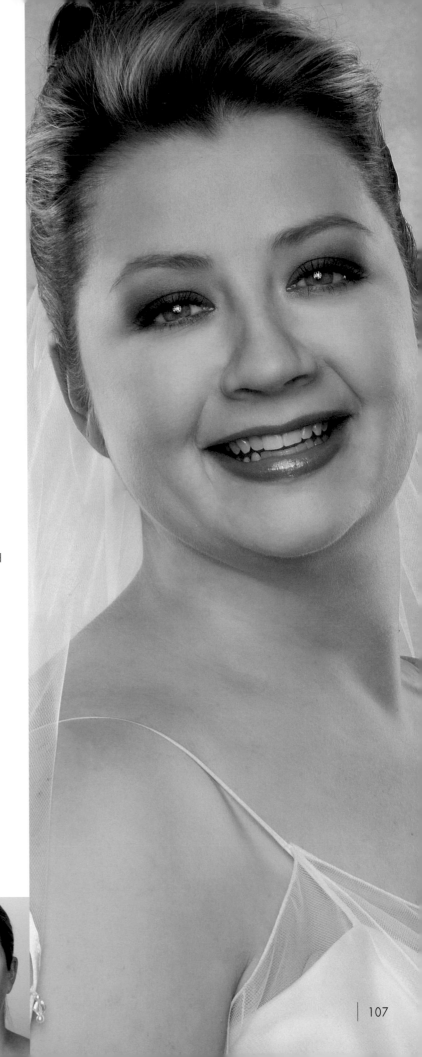

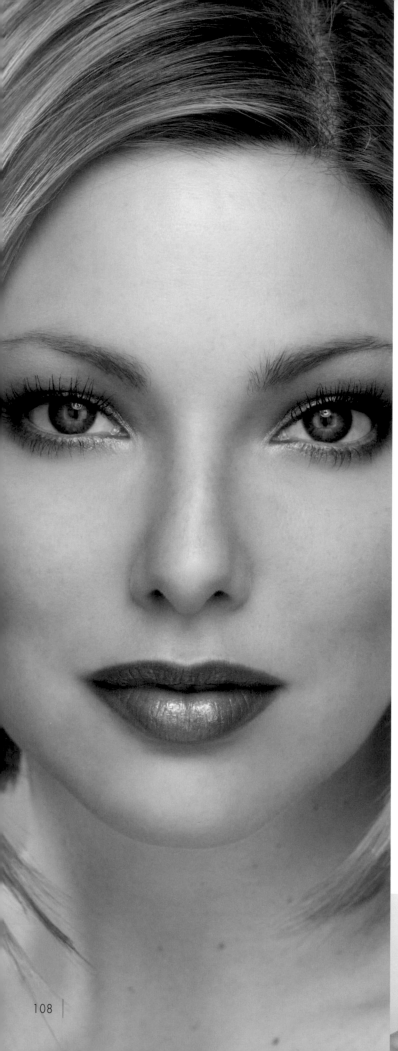

kate

WEDDING TIME:	morning/midday/ late afternoon/evening
EYESHADOW APPLICATION:	sparkling eye (page 84)
EYESHADOW:	highlight: matte nude/ shimmer flesh midtone: matte taupe contour: matte mahogany
BLUSH:	rich honey
LIP LINER:	deep coral
LIPSTICK:	warm pink
LIP GLOSS:	shimmer coral
TIPS:	To make the shimmer highlight eyeshadow shade show the most, I first layered a matte nude color on the lid (to create a base), then applied the shimmer highlight eyeshadow shade on top to make it stand out even more. I chose not to use any eyeliner, and instead got all my lash definition from using contour eyeshadow shade all along the lashline along with lots of thick dark lashes. This is such a great look because it works at any time of day!

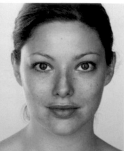

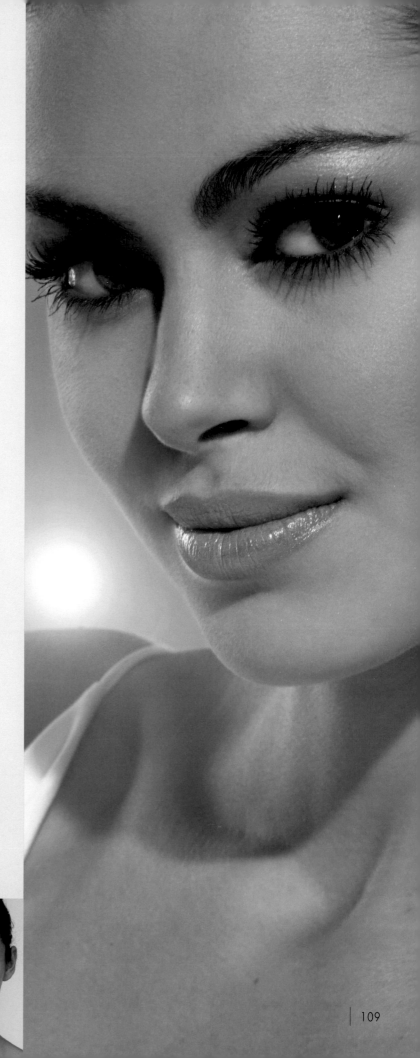

nonna

WEDDING TIME:	morning/midday/late afternoon
EYESHADOW APPLICATION:	sparkling eye (page 84)
EYESHADOW:	highlight: shimmer gold midtone: matte caramel blush: rich honey
LIP LINER:	flesh
LIPSTICK:	pinkish nude
LIP GLOSS:	creamy nude
TIPS:	I wanted a soft monochromatic look, so I used varying degrees of the same colors. To make the eyes even more subtle, I only used a highlight and midtone, and didn't use any eyeliner. In order to get more eye definition, I simply defined the lashline with the midtone eyeshadow shade and thick dark lashes. To continue the subtle monochromatic look, I used subtle cheek and lip color in the same shade family. Overall, this treatment gives you a soft, natural, glowing look!

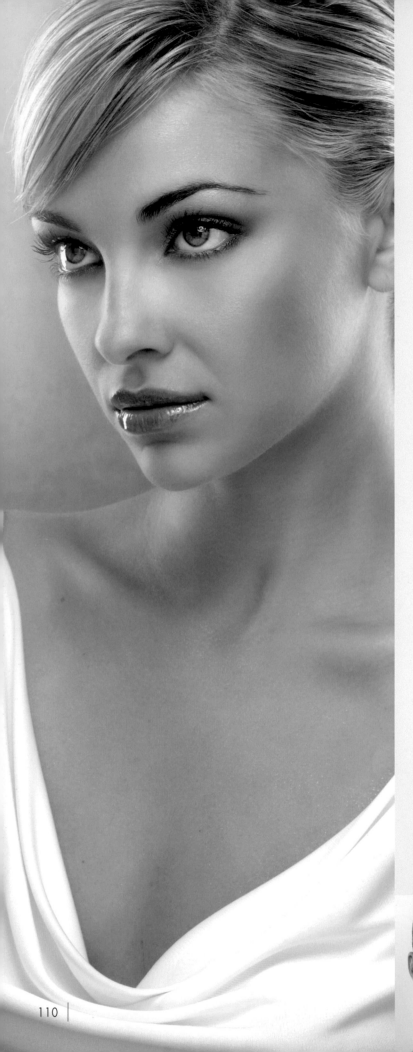

glenna

WEDDING TIME:	morning/midday/ late afternoon/evening
EYESHADOW APPLICATION:	natural beauty (page 79)
EYESHADOW:	highlight: shimmer flesh midtone: matte taupe contour: shimmer golden brown
EYELINER:	bronze
BLUSH:	soft peach
LIP LINER:	flesh
LIPSTICK:	pinkish nude
LIP GLOSS:	shimmer coral
TIPS:	You can never go wrong with subtle beauty when it comes to a bride. For Glenna, I chose soft, warm, natural shades from eyes to lips. I have created definition without overpowering her own true beauty!

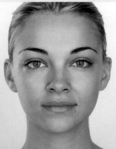

fabiana

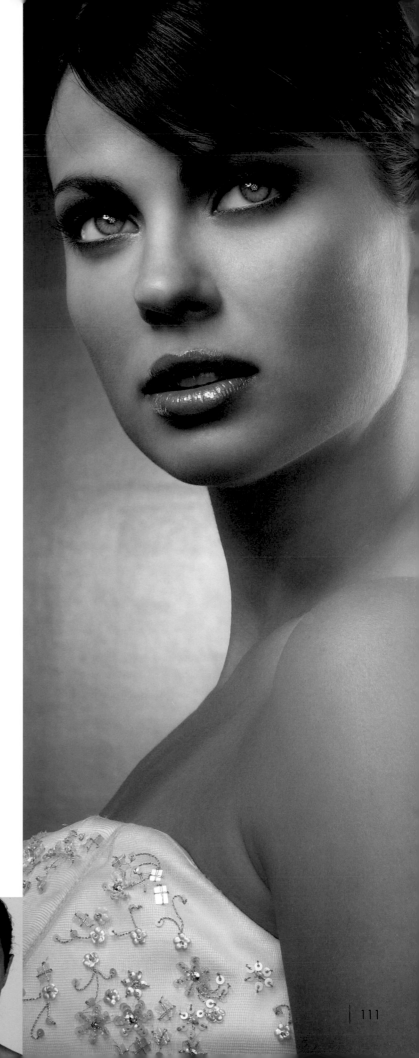

WEDDING TIME:	late afternoon/evening
EYESHADOW APPLICATION:	natural beauty (page 79)
EYESHADOW:	highlight: shimmer flesh
	midtone: matte taupe
	contour: shimmer golden brown
EYELINER:	rich brown
BLUSH:	rich honey
LIP LINER:	fleshy pink
LIPSTICK:	warm pink
LIP GLOSS:	shimmer berry
TIPS:	Because I have chosen a bit richer lip color, it pushes this look to late afternoon and evening. If I lightened the lip color up a bit and used a little less eyeshadow contour color, this look could work at any time of day. But of course I wanted drama!

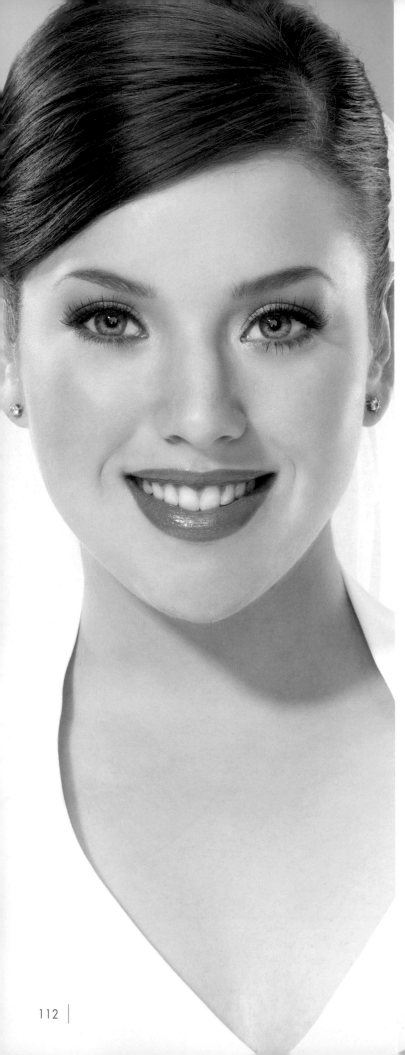

joy

WEDDING TIME:	midday/late afternoon/evening
EYESHADOW APPLICATION:	natural beauty (page 79)
EYESHADOW:	highlight: shimmer gold midtone: matte taupe contour: shimmer chocolate
EYELINER:	bronze
BLUSH:	soft peach
LIP LINER:	deep coral
LIPSTICK:	soft peach
LIP GLOSS:	shimmer coral
TIPS:	Yes, this is our cover girl, and for Joy I went for total glamour. Joy is our resident sweet, adorable diva, and I wanted to make sure she was the center of the universe on her special day. I chose very natural shades, and applied them with a bit more intensity for a little more drama. This look would be perfect for any bride, but more importantly, it is the perfect look for "Princess Joy!"

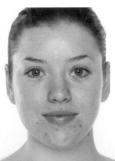

susan

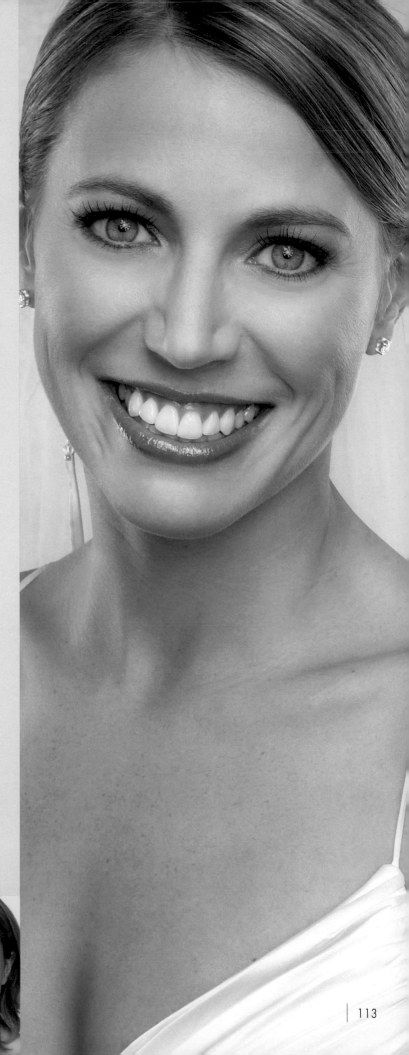

WEDDING TIME:	morning/midday/ late afternoon/evening
EYESHADOW APPLICATION:	natural beauty (page 79)
EYESHADOW:	highlight: shimmer flesh midtone: matte taupe contour: shimmer golden brown
EYELINER:	bronze
BLUSH:	warm pink
LIP LINER:	warm caramel
LIPSTICK:	soft peach
LIP GLOSS:	shimmer warm pink
TIPS:	Choosing subtle, natural shades will always make a look work at any time of day. Here, I made sure to (as always) bronze first, then I chose a blush that would give Susan's face a soft, flushed glow. Pretty skin always makes a pretty picture!

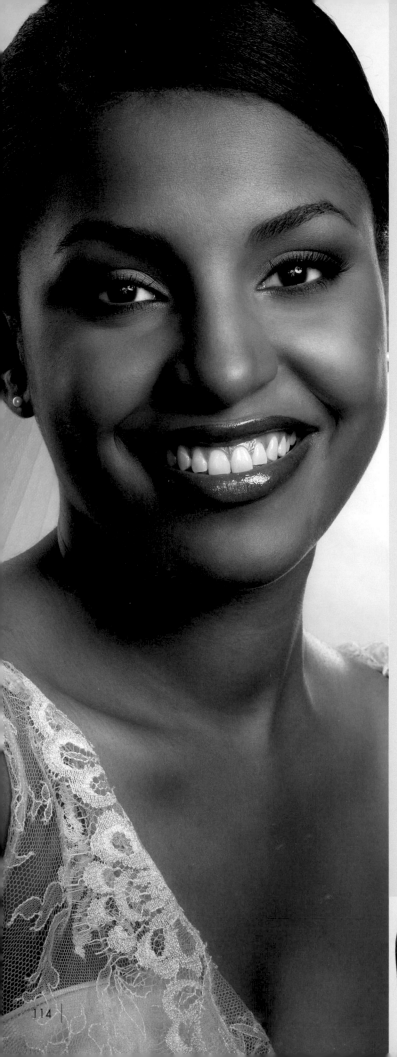

kim

WEDDING TIME:	late afternoon/evening
EYESHADOW APPLICATION:	natural beauty (page 79)
EYESHADOW:	highlight: matte sand midtone: matte mahogany contour: matte charcoal
EYELINER:	charcoal
BLUSH:	rich terracotta
LIP LINER:	warm caramel
LIPSTICK:	golden nude
LIP GLOSS:	shimmer berry
TIPS:	I went a bit more dramatic for Kim's look. I chose a very intense eyeshadow contour color so that the attention would be on her eyes. Of course, with eyes that are a bit more dramatic like this, I made sure that her lip color was very subtle, choosing to get all the color from the gloss and not the lipstick.

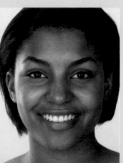

tiffany

WEDDING TIME:	morning/midday/ late afternoon/evening
EYESHADOW APPLICATION:	natural beauty (page 79)
EYESHADOW:	highlight: shimmer flesh midtone: matte dark taupe contour: shimmer chocolate
EYELINER:	rich brown
BLUSH:	rich honey
LIP LINER:	flesh
LIPSTICK:	soft peach
LIP GLOSS:	shimmer warm pink
TIPS:	Talk about a princess! Tiffany could get married at any time of day with her look. (It is never wrong to wear a tiara!) I really gave her skin a lot of color and glow with bronzer. By adding a bit of color and depth to the skin, I made sure it will photograph beautifully, even in the evening with a flash.

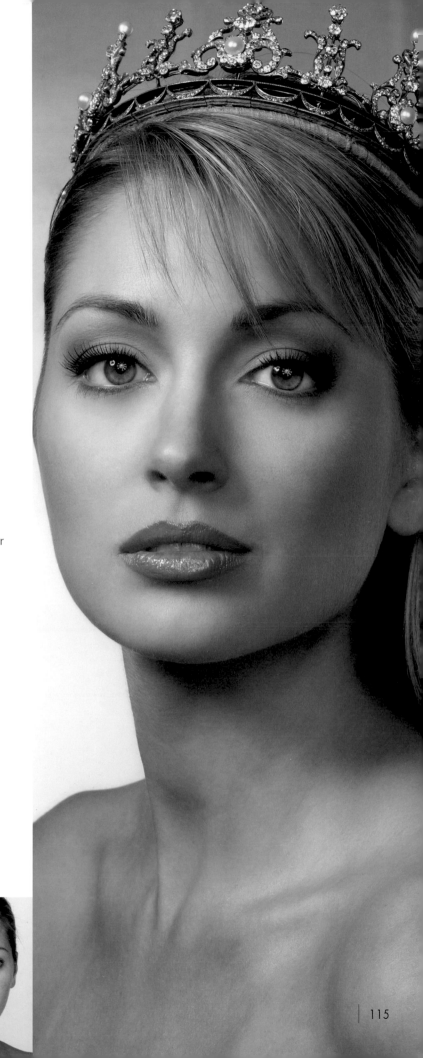

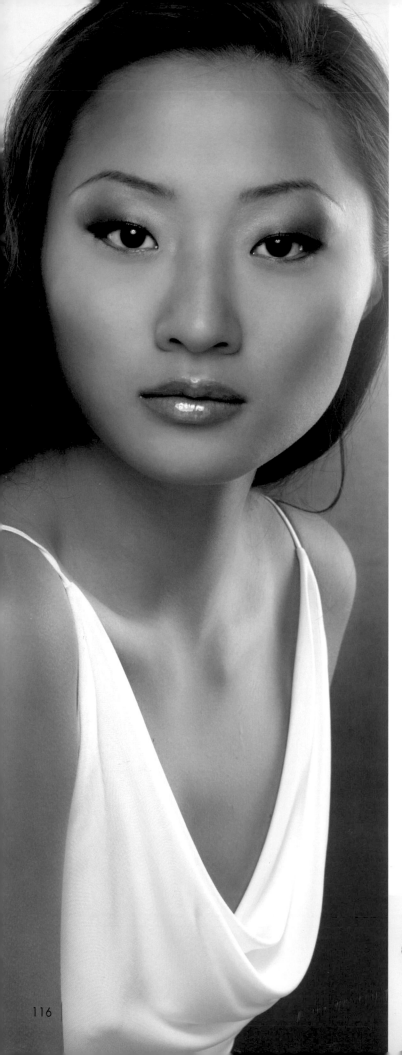

sylvia

WEDDING TIME:	late afternoon/evening
EYESHADOW APPLICATION:	natural beauty (page 79)
EYESHADOW:	highlight: shimmer beige midtone: matte taupe contour: matte dark brown
EYELINER:	rich brown
BLUSH:	rich honey
LIP LINER:	flesh
LIPSTICK:	pinkish nude
LIP GLOSS:	shimmer coral
TIPS:	Normally, a look like Sylvia's would have also worked for midday, but I chose to apply a contour eyeshadow shade with more intensity, so this look works better in the late afternoon or evening. Also, since I intensified the eyes, I kept the cheeks and lips subtle.

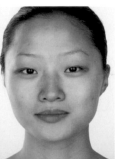

alyssa

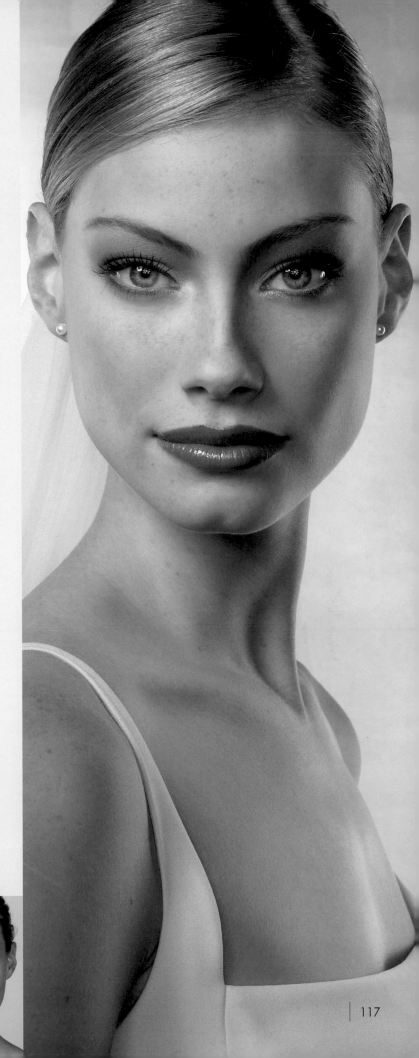

WEDDING TIME:	morning/midday/ late afternoon/evening
EYESHADOW APPLICATION:	natural beauty (page 79)
EYESHADOW:	highlight: shimmer flesh midtone: matte taupe contour: shimmer golden brown
EYELINER:	bronze
BLUSH:	soft apricot
LIP LINER:	warm caramel
LIPSTICK:	warm pink
LIP GLOSS:	shimmer coral
TIPS:	Alyssa's look works at any time of day because of its soft, subtle application and shade choices. Sometimes it is just as beautiful *not* to draw attention to any one feature on the face. Instead, choose shades that will give the same amount of soft, subtle definition to all your features.

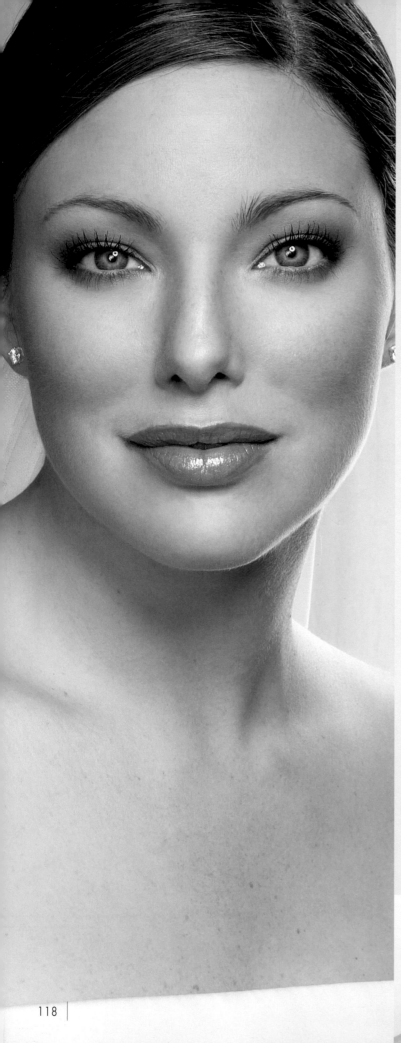

kate

WEDDING TIME:	morning/midday/ late afternoon/evening
EYESHADOW APPLICATION:	natural beauty (page 79)
EYESHADOW:	highlight: shimmer flesh midtone: matte taupe contour: shimmer golden brown
BLUSH:	rich honey
LIP LINER:	flesh
LIPSTICK:	pinkish nude
LIP GLOSS:	shimmer coral
TIPS:	What can I say, other than this is the perfect balance of beauty and definition? I've brought out every feature, without one feature overpowering another. I also chose not to use eyeliner. Instead, I simply used my contour eyeshadow shade to define Kate's eyes all along the lashline. And don't forget thick, gorgeous lashes!

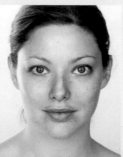

poppi

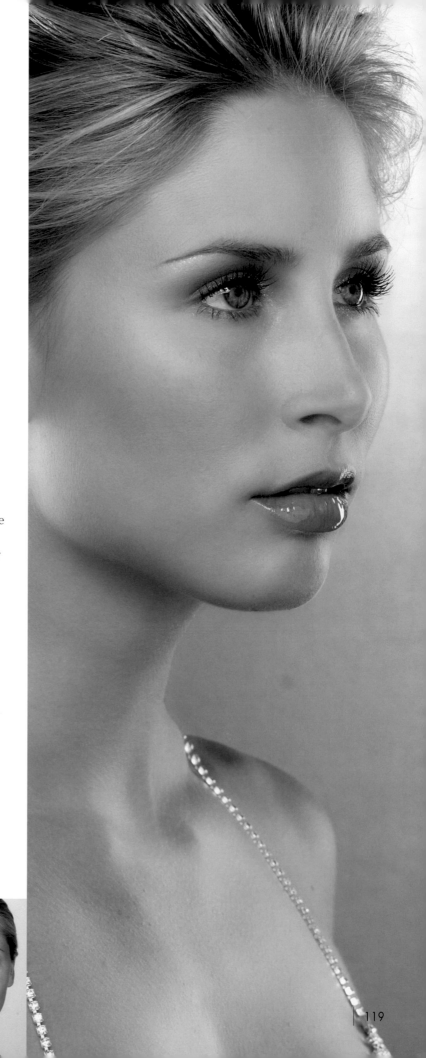

WEDDING TIME:	morning/midday/late afternoon
EYESHADOW APPLICATION:	sparkling eye (page 84)
EYESHADOW:	highlight: matte nude/ shimmer beige midtone: matte rose contour: matte dark taupe
BLUSH:	warm pink
LIP LINER:	flesh
LIPSTICK:	warm pink
LIP GLOSS:	creamy nude
TIPS:	To make the shimmer highlight eyeshadow shade show the most, I first layered a matte nude color on the lid (to create a base), then applied the shimmer highlight eyeshadow shade on top to make it stand out even more. To keep this look the ultimate in natural, I chose not to use any eyeliner. I simply defined the lashline with the contour eyeshadow shade and thick, dark lashes.

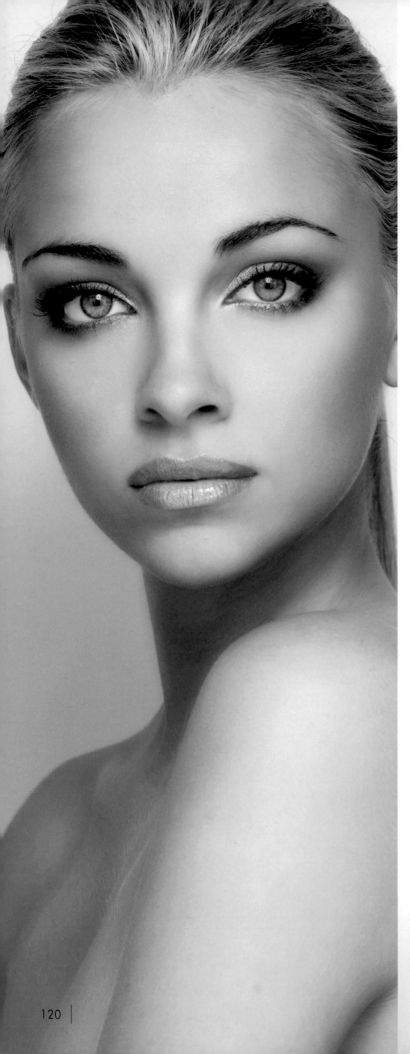

glenna

WEDDING TIME:	late afternoon/evening
EYESHADOW APPLICATION:	natural beauty (page 79)
EYESHADOW:	highlight: shimmer flesh midtone: matte taupe contour: shimmer purple
EYELINER:	purple
BLUSH:	soft peach
LIP LINER:	flesh
LIPSTICK:	pinkish nude
LIP GLOSS:	creamy nude
TIPS:	Okay, I couldn't stand it any longer! I needed a little fun and color. However, adding some color to Glenna's palette limits what times of day her look is appropriate. This look is definitely for a bride who is a glamour girl and wants to play with color.

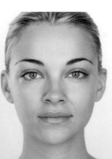

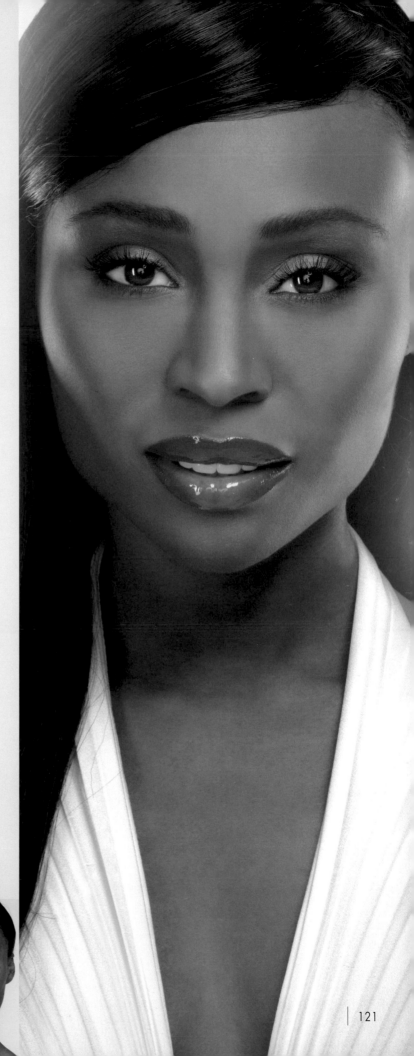

cynthia

WEDDING TIME:	late afternoon/evening
EYESHADOW APPLICATION:	natural beauty (page 79)
EYESHADOW:	highlight: shimmer gold midtone: matte mahogany contour: shimmer purple
EYELINER:	charcoal
BLUSH:	rich terracotta
LIP LINER:	warm caramel
LIPSTICK:	golden nude
LIP GLOSS:	creamy nude
TIPS:	Drama, drama, drama—sometimes it is the only way to go! This is a look Cynthia can definitely pull off. I just want to remind you that whenever you're creating a dramatic eye look, you always want to keep the lips soft and natural. And it never hurts to make them glossy and shiny. You know every man wants to kiss those lips!

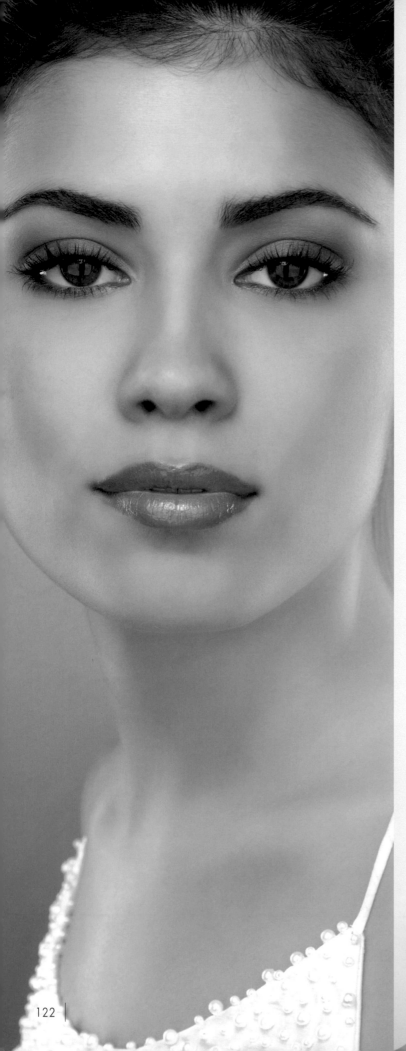

lauren

WEDDING TIME:	evening
EYESHADOW APPLICATION:	smoky eye (page 83)
EYESHADOW:	highlight: shimmer flesh midtone: matte taupe contour: shimmer purple
EYELINER:	purple
BLUSH:	soft apricot
LIP LINER:	flesh
LIPSTICK:	soft peach
LIP GLOSS:	shimmer coral
TIPS:	The bride is supposed to be the center of attention, and Lauren definitely will be! This is a very strong look that I would only do for an evening wedding. I probably would also not choose this look for a blonde, but because of Lauren's coloring, she wears it well.

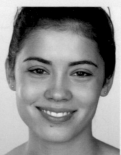

nonna

WEDDING TIME:	evening
EYESHADOW APPLICATION:	smoky eye (page 83)
EYESHADOW:	highlight: shimmer gold
	midtone: matte taupe
	contour: matte charcoal
EYELINER:	charcoal
BLUSH:	warm pink
LIP LINER:	flesh
LIPSTICK:	pinkish nude
LIP GLOSS:	shimmer coral
TIPS:	Nonna's look is the perfect example of a smoky bridal eye. I used simple, natural shades to make it as subtle a look as a smoky eye can be. You get great drama without it being too much. This look is only for the evening bride. Don't forget to choose a soft, natural nude lip for the perfect balance.

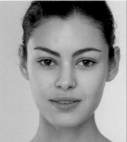

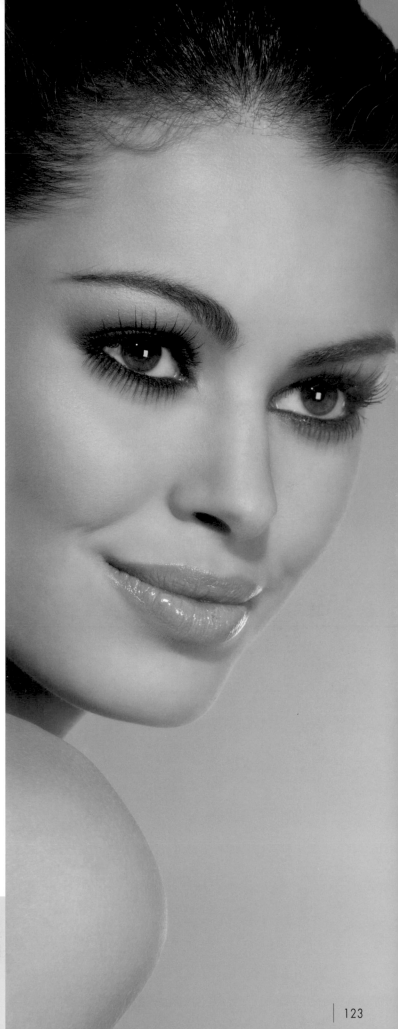

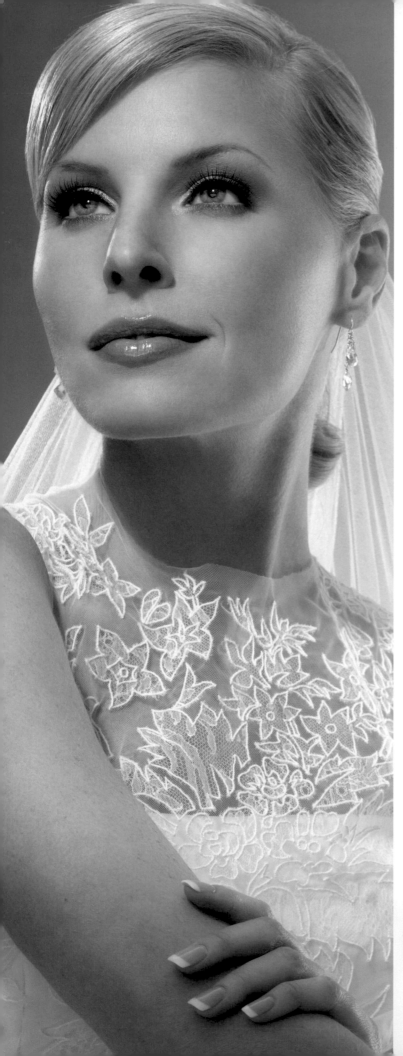

kiley

WEDDING TIME:	late afternoon/evening
EYESHADOW APPLICATION:	sparkling eye (page 84)
EYESHADOW:	highlight: matte nude/ shimmer beige midtone: matte taupe contour: matte mahogany
EYELINER:	rich brown
BLUSH:	warm pink
LIP LINER:	flesh
LIPSTICK:	soft peach
LIP GLOSS:	shimmer coral
TIPS:	To make the shimmer highlight eyeshadow shade show the most, I first layered a matte nude color on the lid (to create a base), then applied the shimmer highlight eyeshadow shade on top to make it stand out even more. I still defined really well at the lashline with liner and thick, dark lashes. Normally, this is a look that works well at midday, but since I chose a bit darker contour eyeshadow shade and a dark liner, it is better for late afternoon or evening.

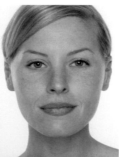

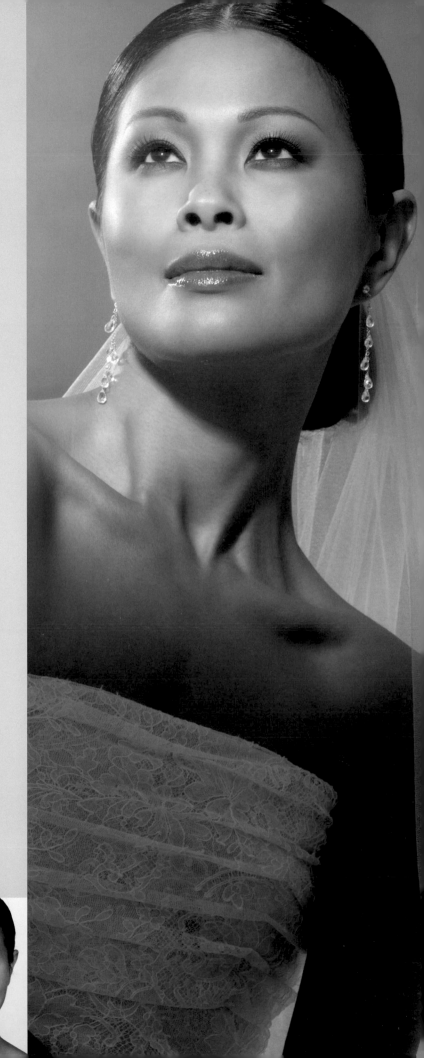

eleanor

WEDDING TIME:	evening
EYESHADOW APPLICATION:	smoky eye (page 83)
EYESHADOW:	highlight: shimmer flesh midtone: matte dark taupe contour: matte mahogany
EYELINER:	rich brown
BLUSH:	rich honey
LIP LINER:	warm caramel
LIPSTICK:	soft peach
LIP GLOSS:	shimmer berry
TIPS:	Glamour was the goal of the day, and I achieved it. I chose a smoky eye with rich, subtle color to create a look that everyone will notice. By not choosing eyeshadow shades that are too dark, we get the drama without it being overpowering. I needed a subtle lip look because of the dramatic eyes, but I wanted a touch of color, so I used a soft natural lipstick, then layered a sheer berry gloss with shimmer on top. This gives the lips a little more depth and color without being too much.

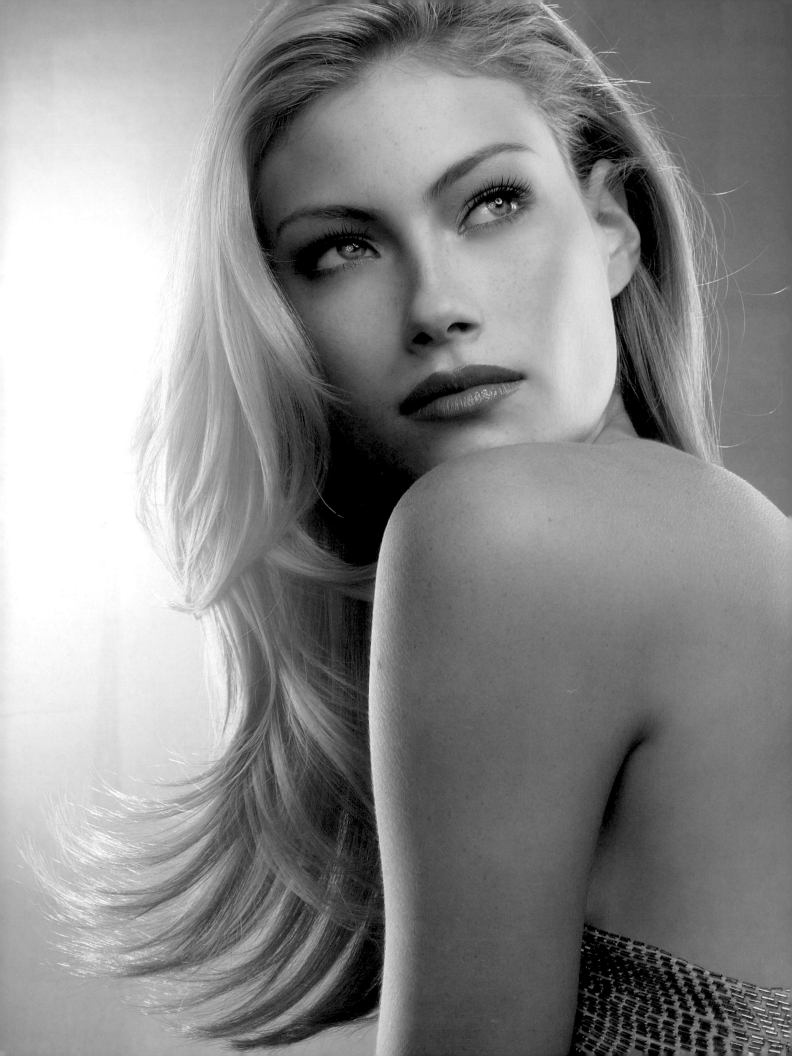

chapter eight | bridesmaids

There are many myths when it comes to makeup looks for bridesmaids. For many years, bridesmaids have been forced to all wear the same makeup colors and shades, no matter what their skin tone. I have looked at so many wedding photos and felt so sorry for all those bridesmaids! First, so often they are made to wear a dress that they never would have picked out for themselves. Then to be forced to wear makeup that is not flattering on top of it. No wonder so many of them end up feeling so unattractive. What a day!

Brides, I appeal to you to have pity on your bridesmaids. Think how *you* would feel in their place! Just as I've shown you how to look beautiful on your special day, I'd like for you to share this chapter with your bridesmaids so they can look and feel beautiful, too. You can all have fun together trying your new makeup looks, and just think how much happier everyone will be! Don't worry—I won't let them upstage you, I promise. After all, it is *your* day!

Let's talk about ways to make your bridesmaids feel beautiful, too. First, as with the bride, we do not want anything too bold or bright, since it will never photograph well. Leaning on the more natural side is the safest and best way to assure beautiful pictures. But you always want to let your bridesmaids feel like themselves. Take into consideration who they are and how they normally wear their makeup—that's what makes them feel beautiful. For the most part, they can still do just that—we just might need to adjust it slightly.

I have some facts and some opinions to share with you. Using this basic information can help create beautiful photographs without stripping each bridesmaid of her individuality. Believe it or not, this can really help your special day flow much more smoothly without unneeded drama. We all know that a woman who feels beautiful is a happy woman.

So here are the facts and a few opinions, of course based on much experience and trial and error.

1. **A bridesmaid's makeup does not have to match her dress.** Makeup is meant to make the girl look more beautiful, not the outfit. Always choose shades that will bring out the girl and her features.

2. **Every girl does not have to wear the same shades of makeup.** There are so many skin tones, we have to consider what each one needs. The only thing that has to match is the intensity of color. You do not want one girl with bold eye makeup and one with almost none. I think a subtle yet defined look always looks good and will photograph perfectly.

3. **Every girl does not have to wear the same shade of lipstick.** I know that this is the most common piece of makeup that everyone thinks just has to match. Once again, the same shade will not look perfect on every girl. The only aspect of the color that has to match is the intensity. You do not want one girl in bold or deep lip color and another in a nude lip color. Once again, a subtle shade that defines yet adds color will always photograph flawlessly.

4. **Have the bride and bridesmaids look the opposite of one another.** This is one thing that I have found really sets the bride apart from the bridesmaids. What I mean by this is: If the bride wears her hair up, all the bridesmaids should wear theirs down. If the bride wears her hair down, all the bridesmaids should wear theirs up. I know this might seem trivial, but in my experience, this makes for beautiful photographs and it helps the bride really stand out.

5. **Most importantly, you never want the bridesmaids' makeup to be more intense than the bride's.** You never want the bridemaids' look to overshadow the bride's! It is her special day, and it is all about her. They are there in a supporting role.

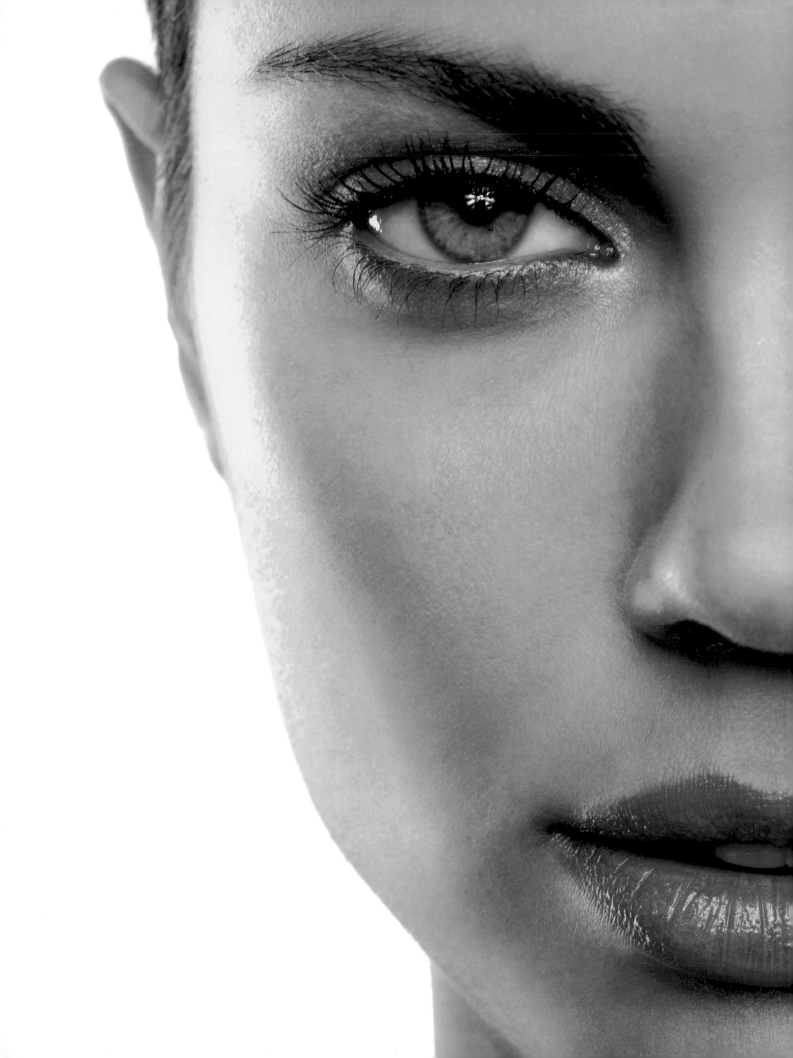

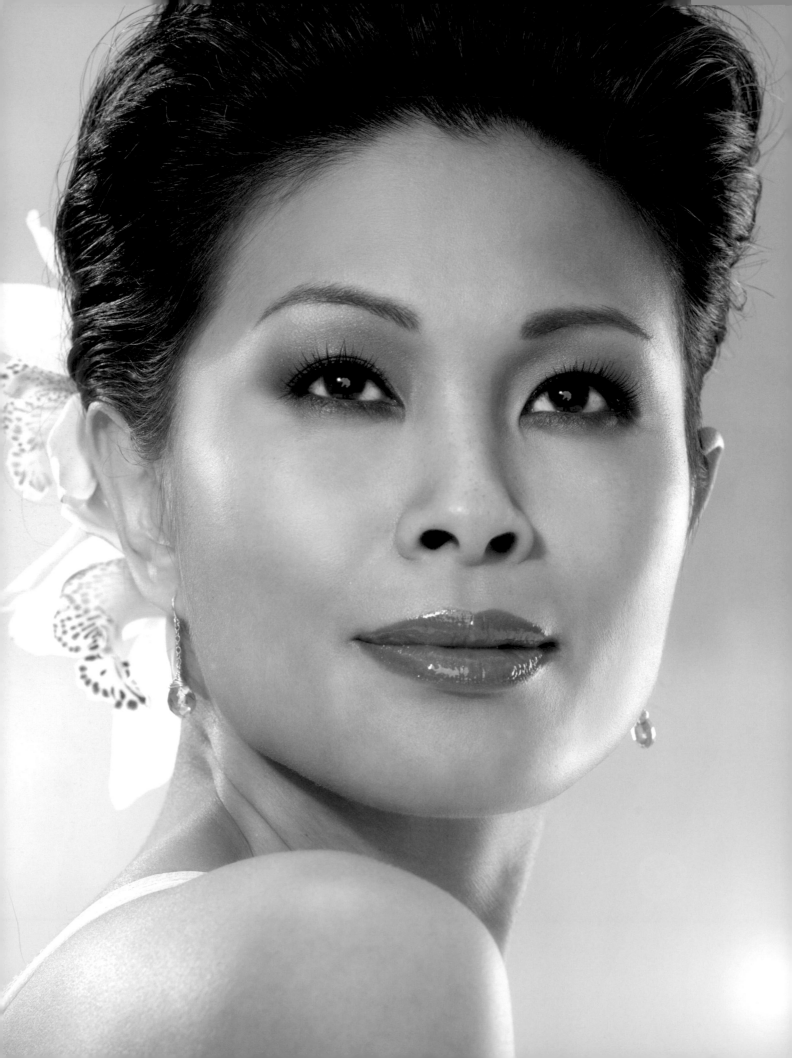

chapter nine | # last but not least

After reading this book, I'm sure you have discovered the best look for your own personal beauty. Everything you have learned is intended to make you feel and look your most beautiful and confident on one of the most special days of your life. If you would like to learn more about the basics of everyday beauty, be sure to look for my book *Makeup Makeovers*.

Makeup Makeovers will demystify the art of makeup by simply explaining products; helping you identifying the best looks for your features; and teaching you simple techniques for applying foundation, eyeshadow, blush, lipstick, and concealer. It is the best handbook for every question you might have about makeup and all the ways you can use it to look your most beautiful.

Most of the tools mentioned in this book are available on my Web site, www.simplebeaute.com, and I have all my favorite makeup accessories available there as well.

I also want to remind you how important it is to remember that makeup is meant to be beautiful, and beautiful makeup is all about the colors you choose and where you place them—not about how much you put on!

Makeup is meant to accentuate and highlight your best features. Instead of focusing on your flaws, learn how to focus on your best features. Remember that every woman is beautiful, and the sooner you discover and celebrate your own personal beauty, the happier and more confident you'll be, whether you're walking down the aisle soon or getting ready for the rest of your life.

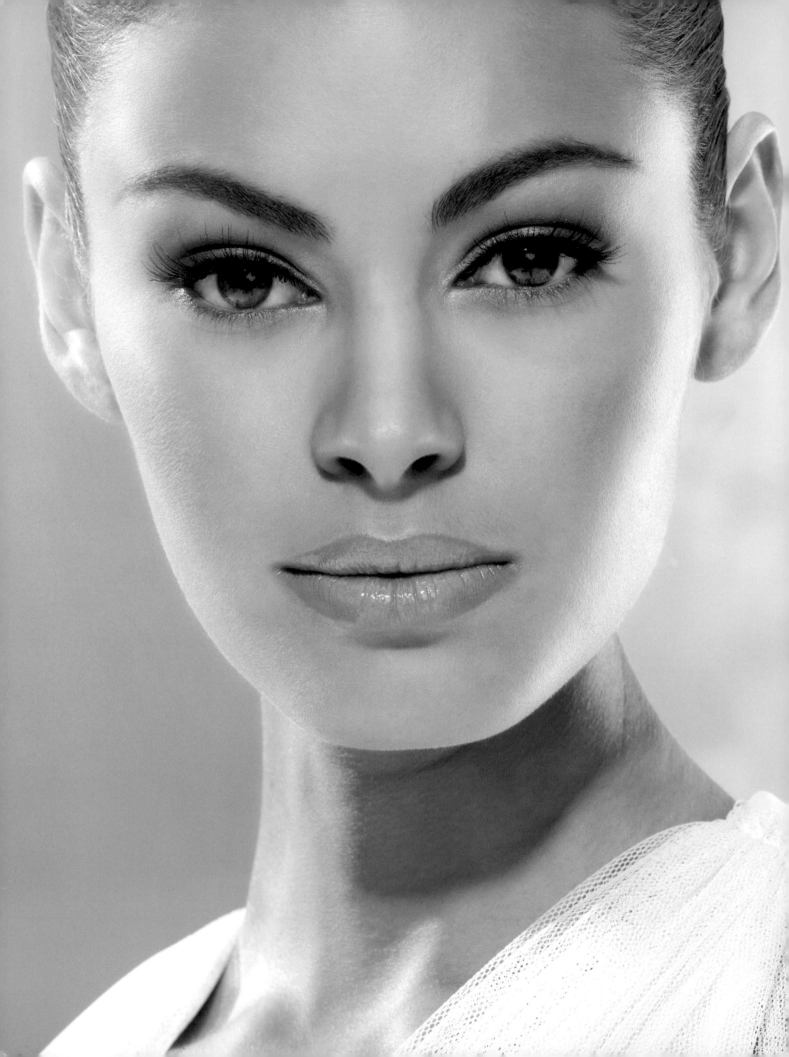

ABOUT THE AUTHOR

Beauty expert Robert Jones, founder of simple beauté, is a respected international hair and makeup artist. Formally trained as a painter at the Houston Museum of Fine Arts, he brings an artist's eye to his work, applying the rules of light, undertones, and blending to some of the world's most recognizable faces.

Robert's work can be found on the pages of *Marie Claire, Allure, In Style, Jane, Elle, Shape, Elegant Bride, Modern Bride,* and numerous other fashion catalogs and magazines. He has traveled the world working on magazine shoots and with numerous celebrities, from rock stars to actresses. He also has had the privilege of working on exciting and lavish celebrity weddings.

Robert's commercial clients include Mary Kay Inc., Neiman Marcus, Bergdorf Goodman, Lord and Taylor, Watters and Watters, and many others. He is the author of *Makeup Makeovers,* a beauty handbook designed to help women of all ages define their best features and build their self-esteem and confidence. He splits his time between New York and Dallas, working on a variety of fashion shoots and commercial projects.

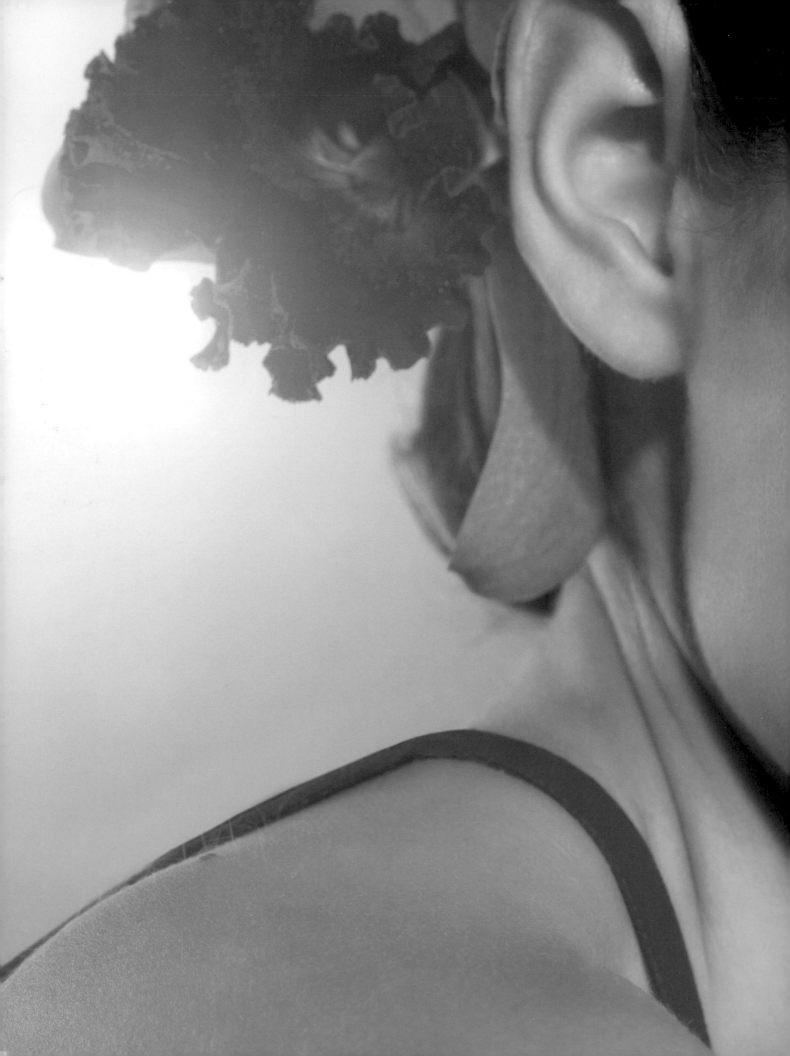

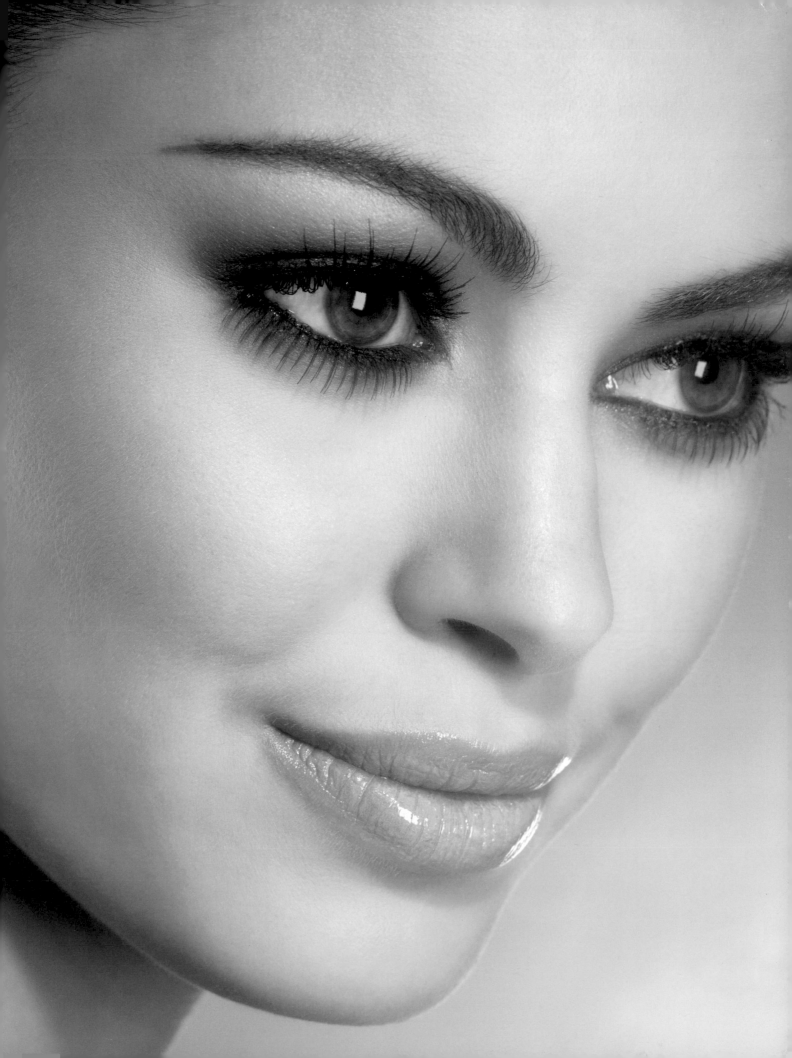

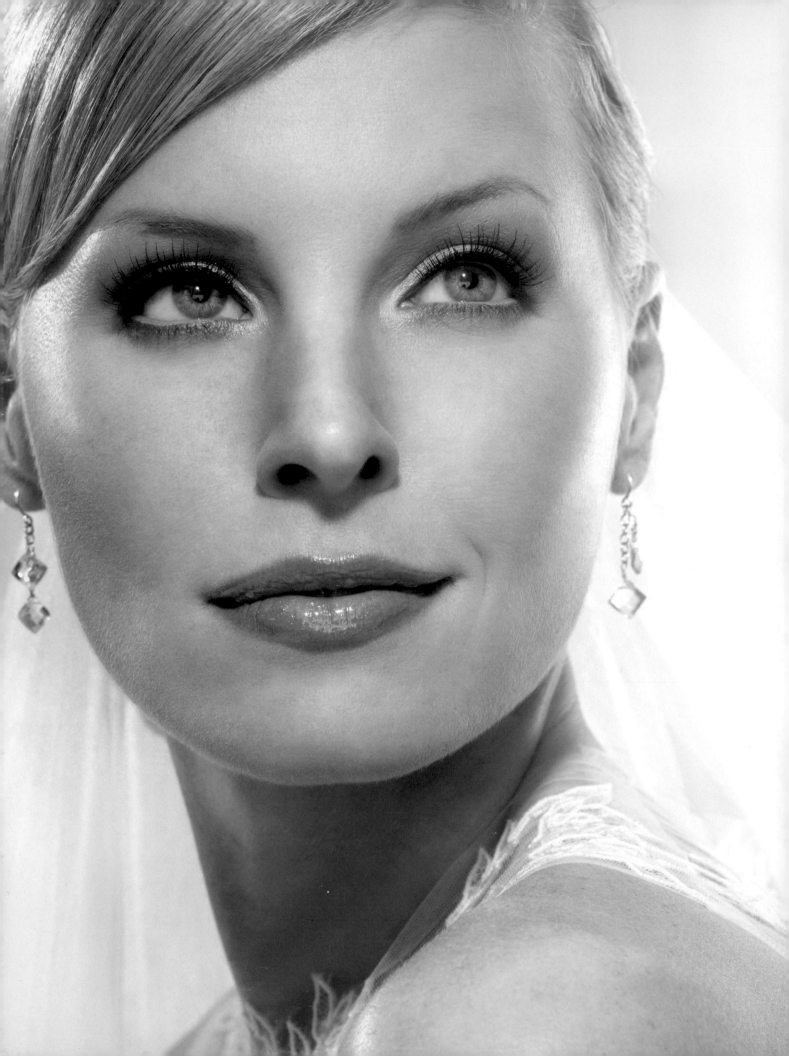